PRESCHOOL
Activity Book
Trucks, Cars, AND Airplanes

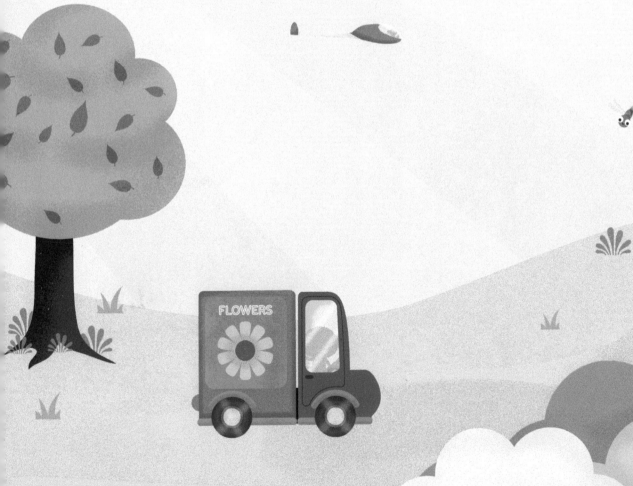

PRESCHOOL Activity Book
Trucks, Cars, AND Airplanes

80 Games to Learn Letters, Numbers, Colors, and Shapes

Valerie Deneen

ILLUSTRATED BY

Rachael McLean

R
ROCKRIDGE
PRESS

NOTE TO PARENTS

Welcome to *Preschool Activity Book: Trucks, Cars, and Airplanes*! This vehicle-themed book includes 80 fun games and activities designed to grab and hold a preschool-aged child's attention and interest. Trucks, planes, boats, and other vehicles are very interesting to young children and are a perfect way to introduce basic early learning skills, such as colors, numbers, letters, words, shapes, and patterns. The activities in each section of the book progress from easiest to hardest. Ones that your child finds easy will help build their confidence. Others that prove to be challenging might be worth skipping and returning to on another day. You should help your child read and follow the directions as needed and make the learning into a fun family activity! Each game can be completed with only crayons, and the book's small size makes it perfect to take with you anywhere. Ready, set, go!

CONTENTS

ANSWER KEY

Ready, Set, Go!

Help the race car speed through the track to get the trophy.

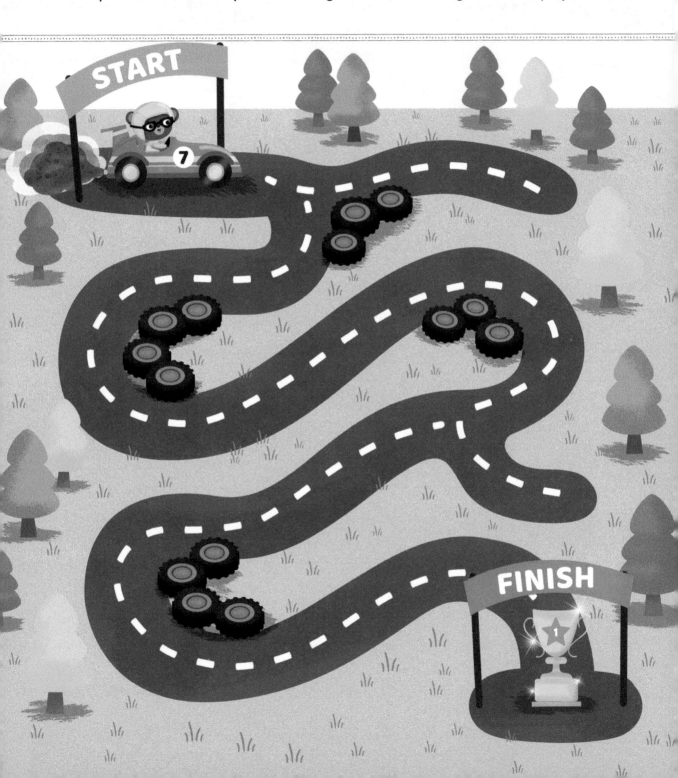

Ride a Wave

Trace the waves that the sailboat is riding on.

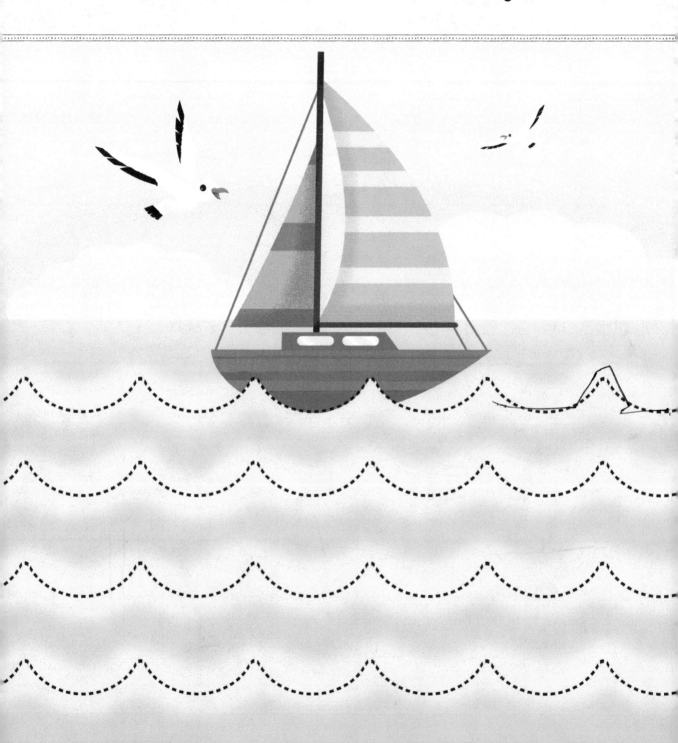

Perfect Parking

Trace the lines to park each car in its garage.

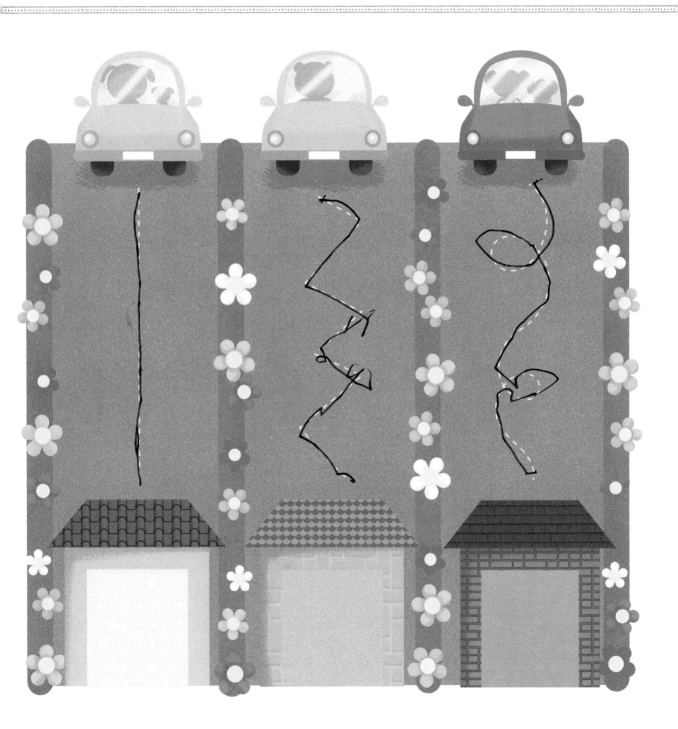

Hospital Helpers

Guide the ambulance to the hospital.

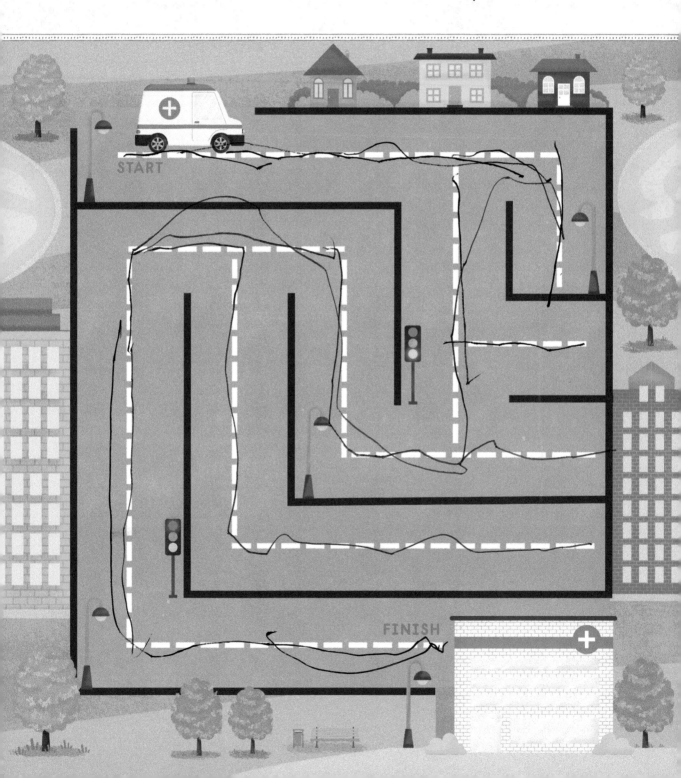

Red Alert

Color 5 of the fire trucks **red**.

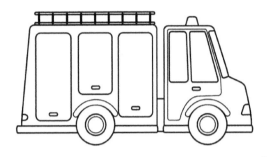
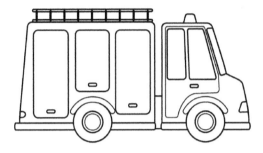
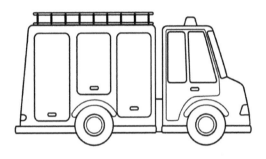
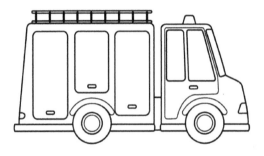
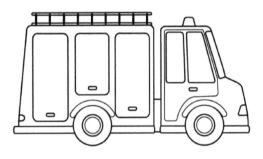
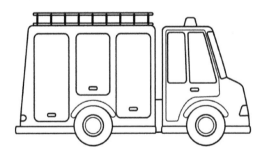
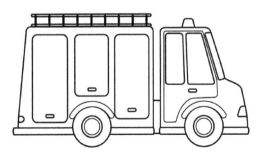
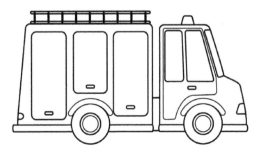

Out of the Blue

Draw an X on all the **blue** things.

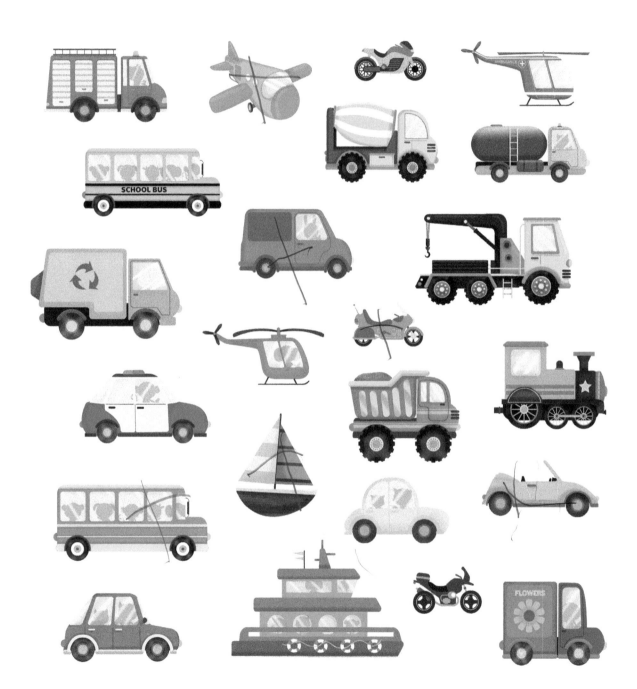

Going Green!

Draw a line to match the green vehicles.

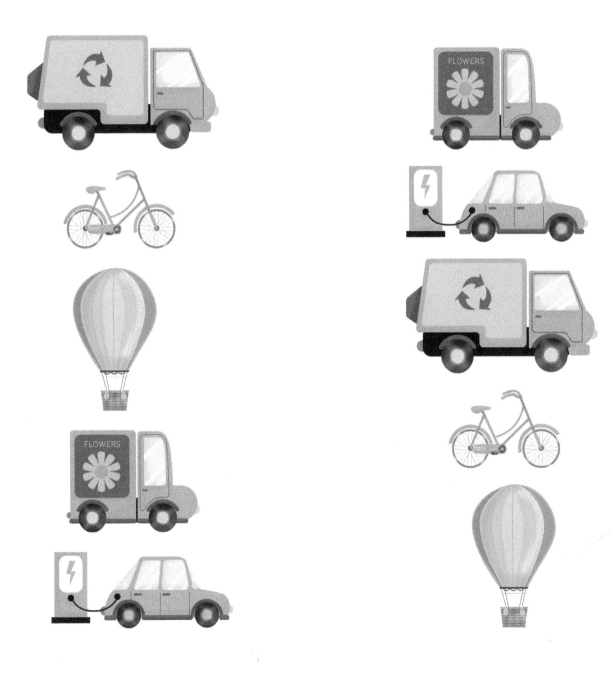

Construction Zone

Trace all the traffic cones and color them orange.

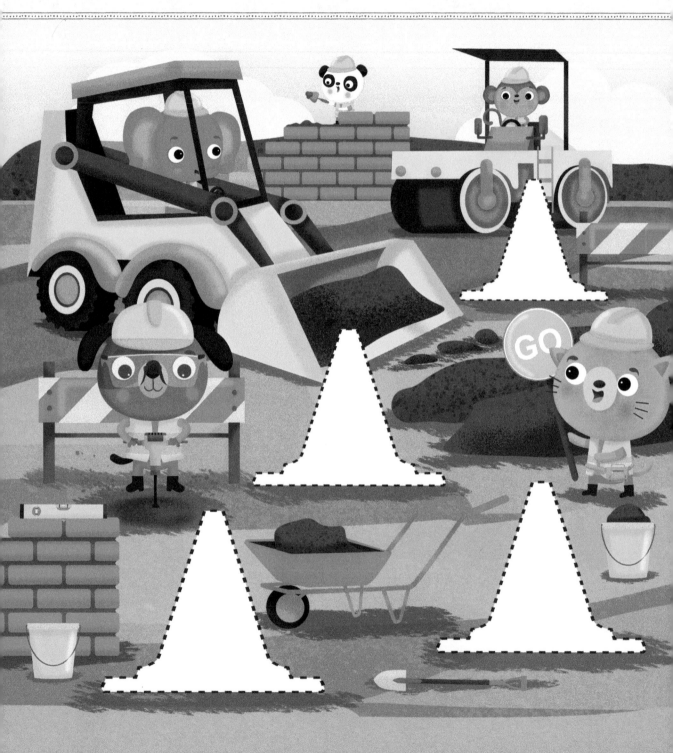

Count & Color

Color the taxis, school buses, and road signs yellow.
How many of each do you see?

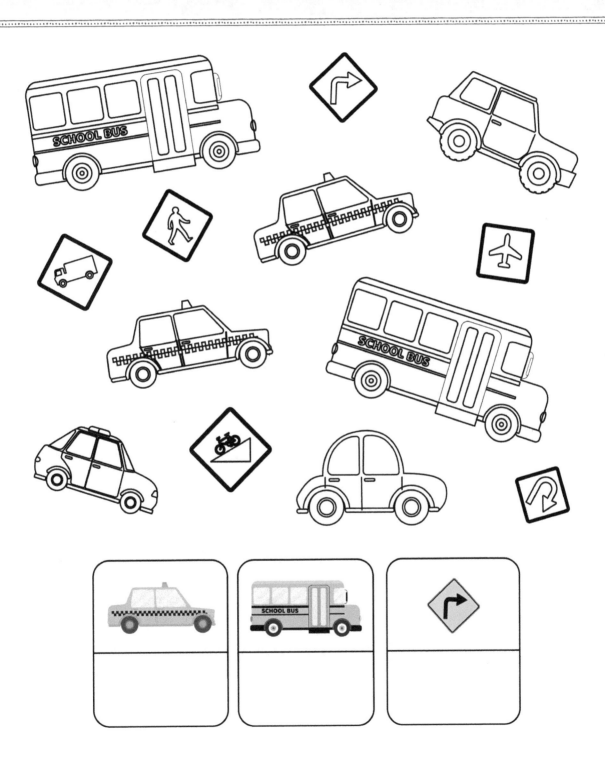

Purple Pickup Trucks

Look closely at both pictures. Find and circle 4 things that are different in the second picture.

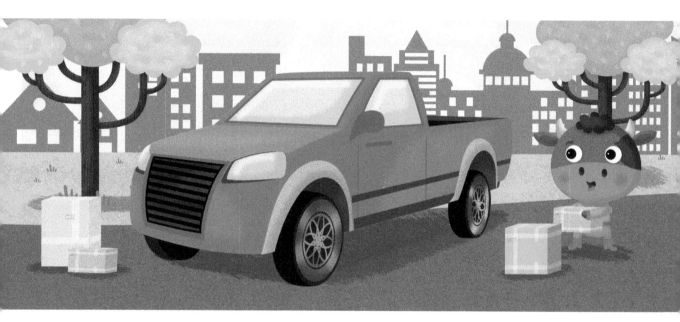

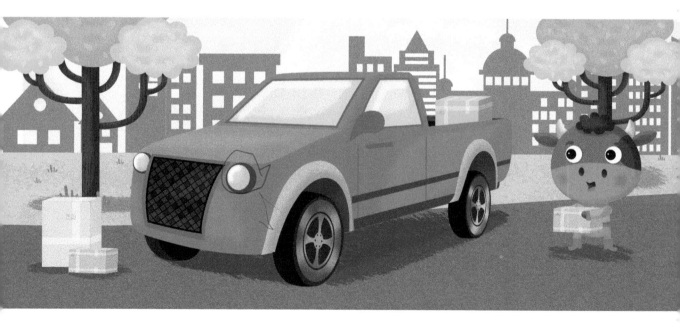

Key to Happiness

Draw a line to match each vehicle with its key.

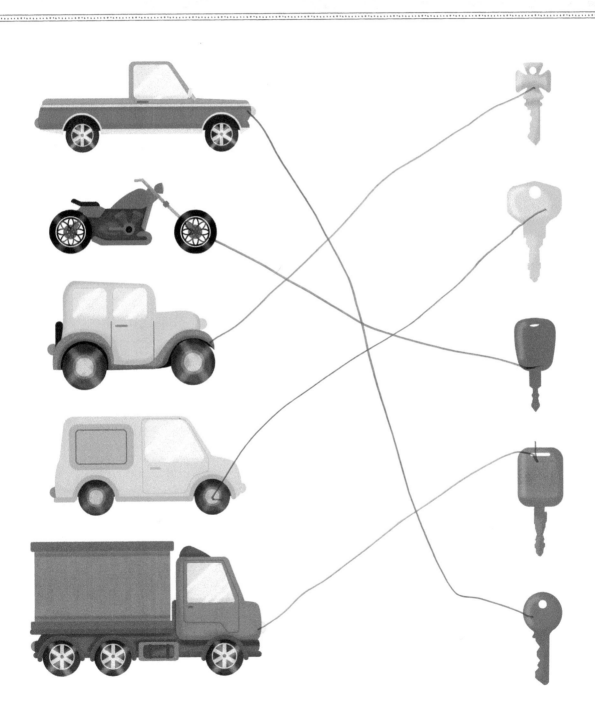

Traffic Jam!

Color the cars **red**, the trucks **green**, and the buses **blue**.

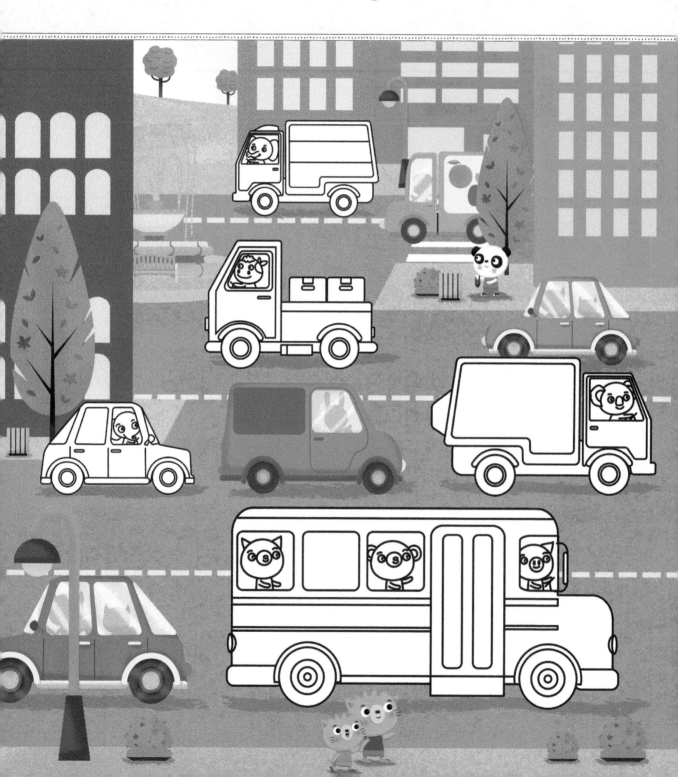

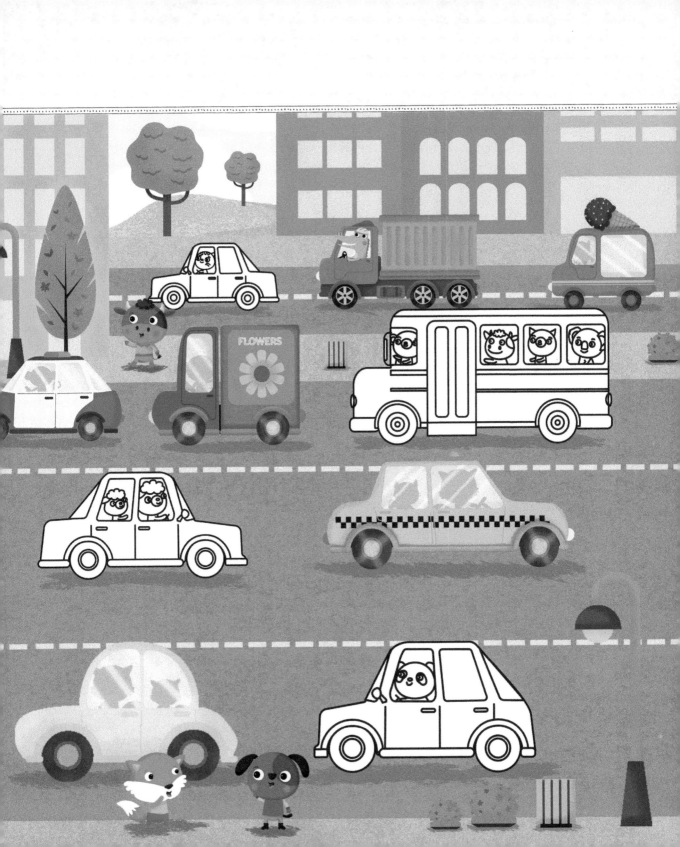

Not So Fast

This speedometer is missing its numbers. Can you trace them?

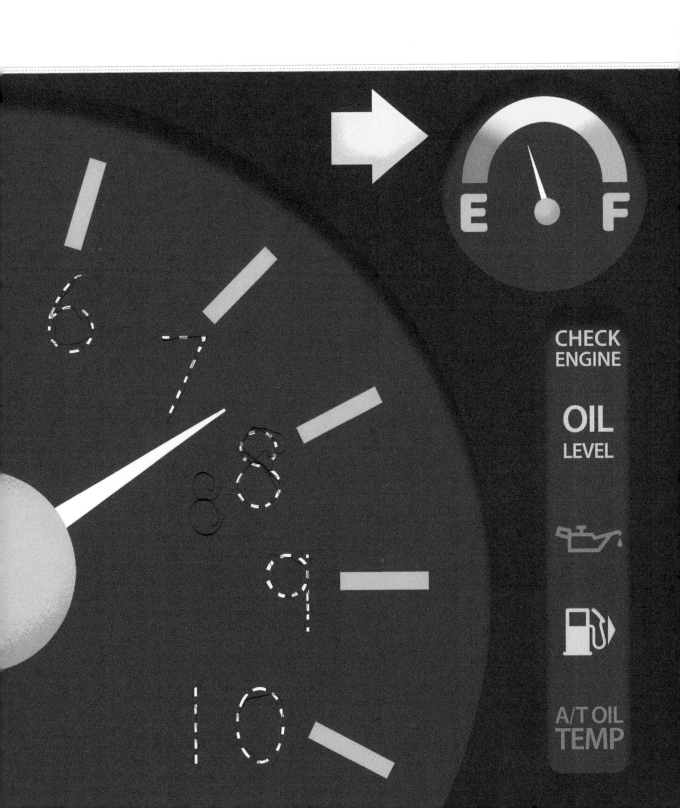

Follow the 1s to get the airplane back to the airport.

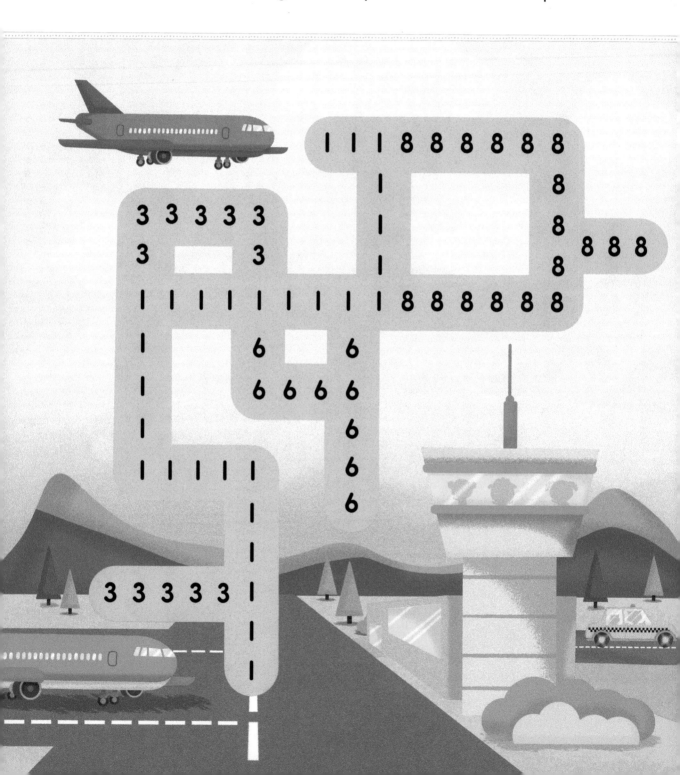

Sailing Away

Color the white sails on the sailboats.
Make them any color you want!

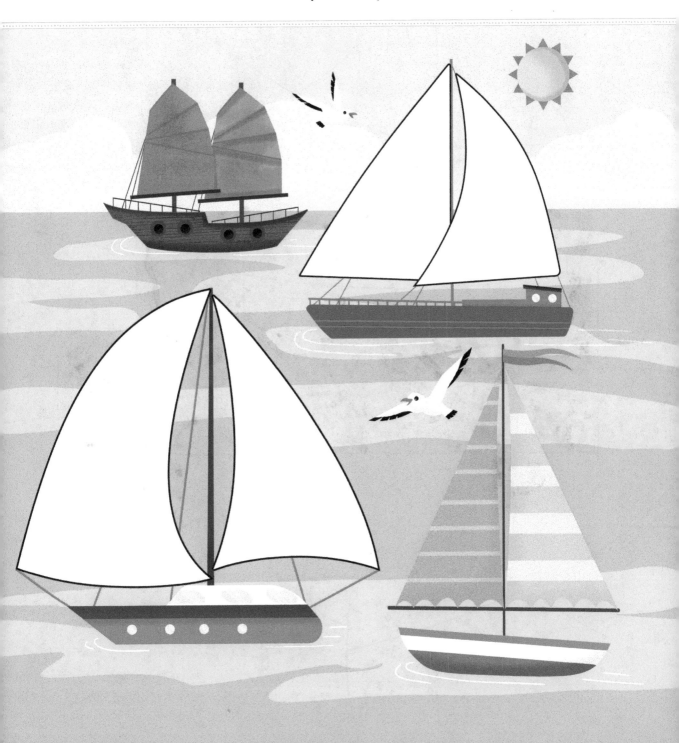

Terrific Two

Color all the spaces with the number 2 yellow.
What do you see?

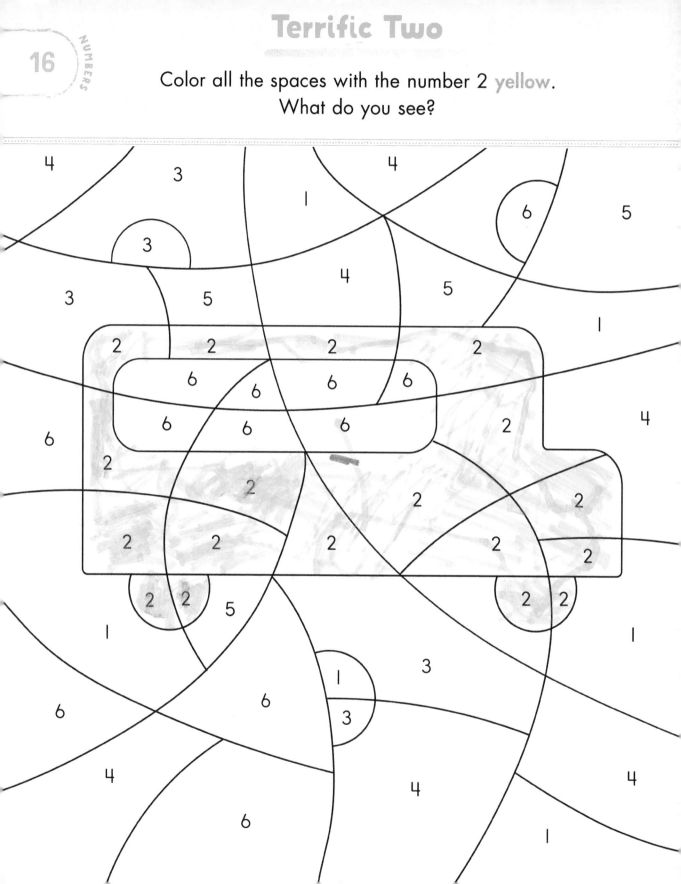

Circle every group that has 3 rescue vehicles in it.

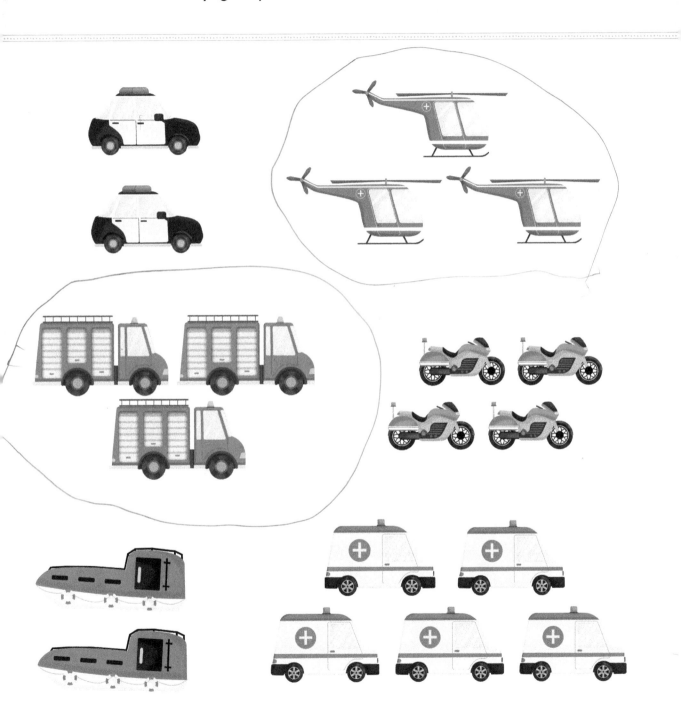

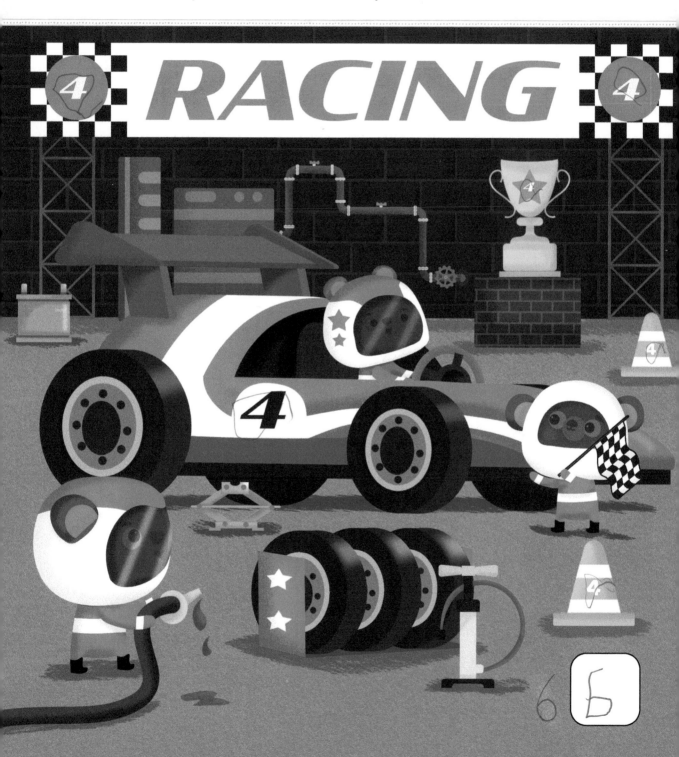

Race Time

How many number 4s can you find hidden
in the picture below? Write your answer in the box.

6

In the Fast Lane

Draw an X on the row with 5 motorcycles.

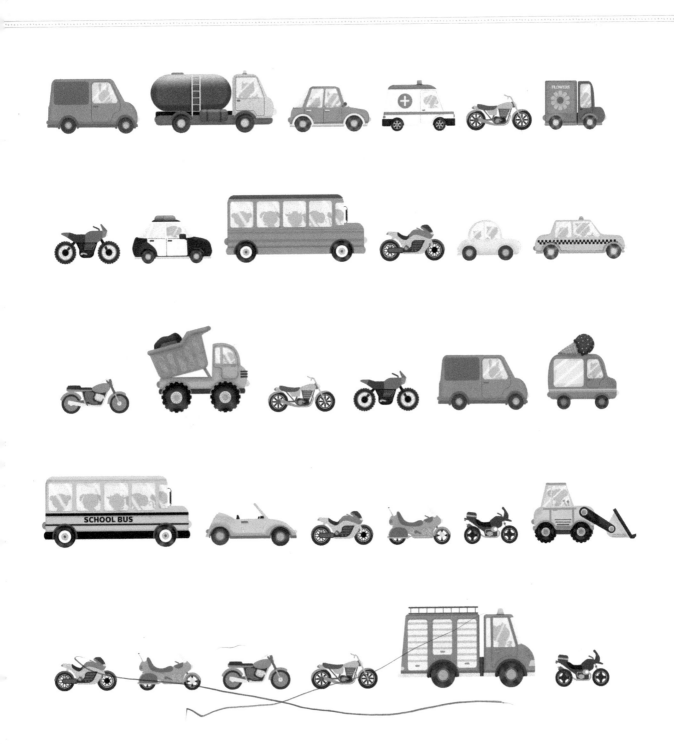

Smooth Sailing

Color all the spaces with the number 6 green.
What do you see?

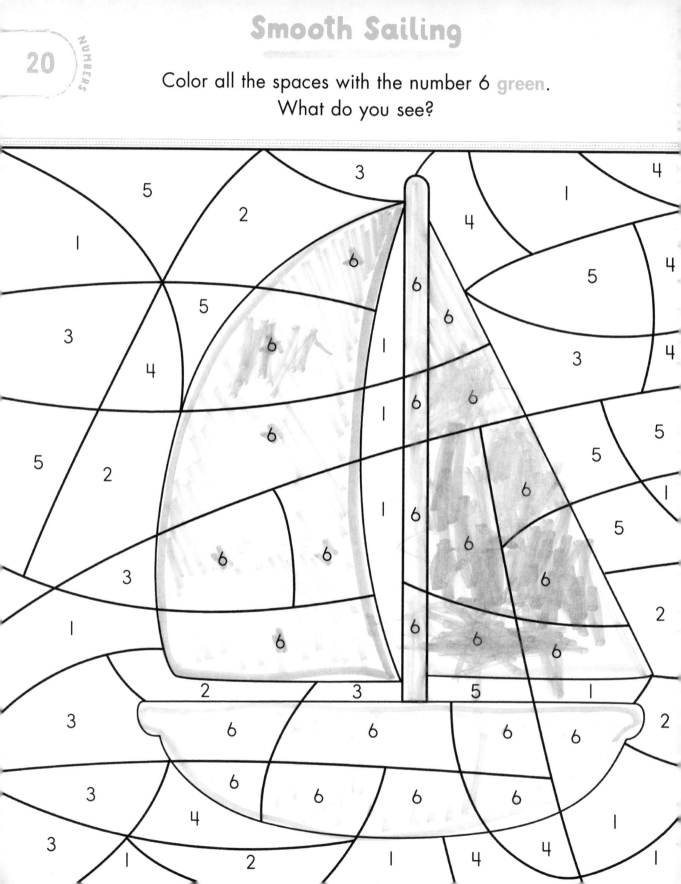

License to Drive

Draw a circle around each license plate that has a 7 as part of its number.

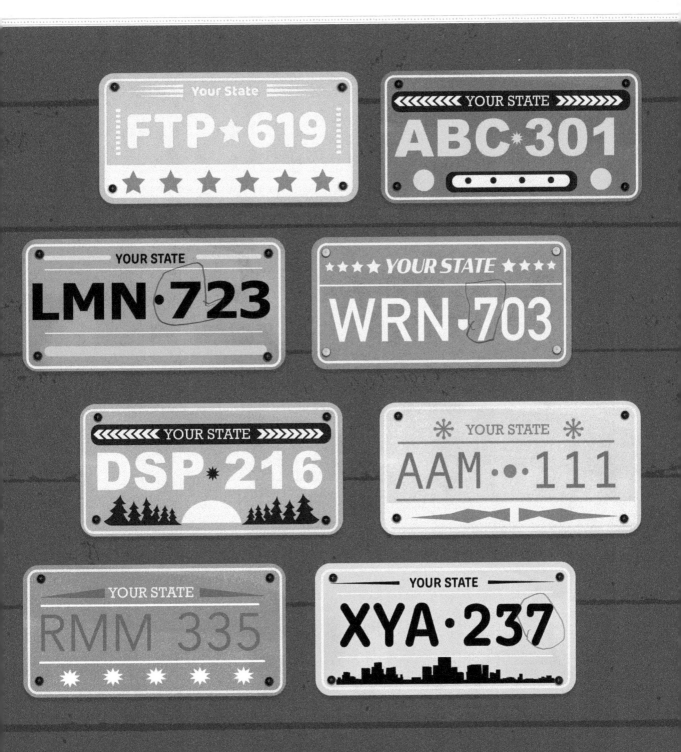

Package Delivery

Follow the 8s to get the mail truck to the post office.

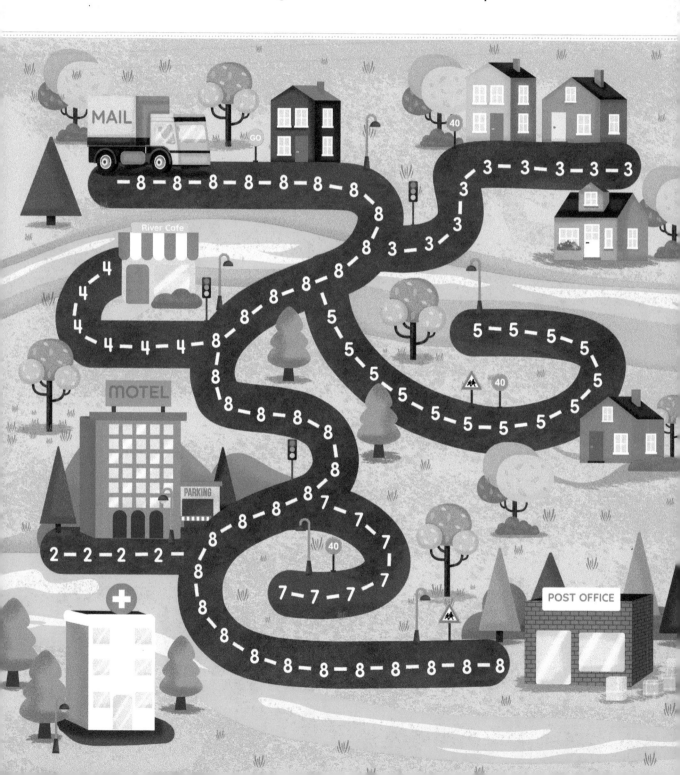

Floating on Air

Color all the spaces with the number 9 **purple**.
What do you see?

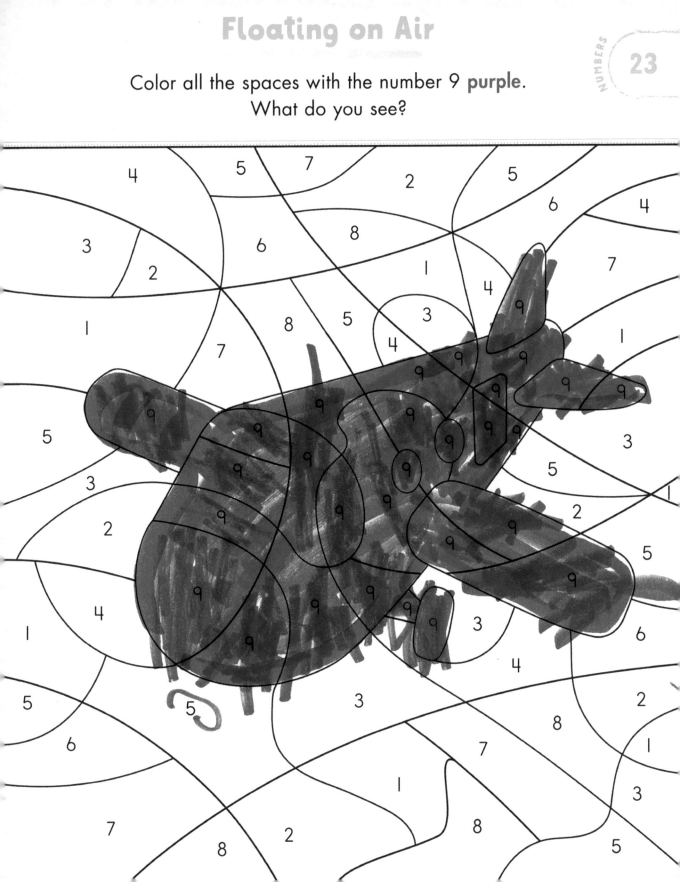

Count on Me

Count the number of vehicles in each row.
Draw a line to match it with the correct number.

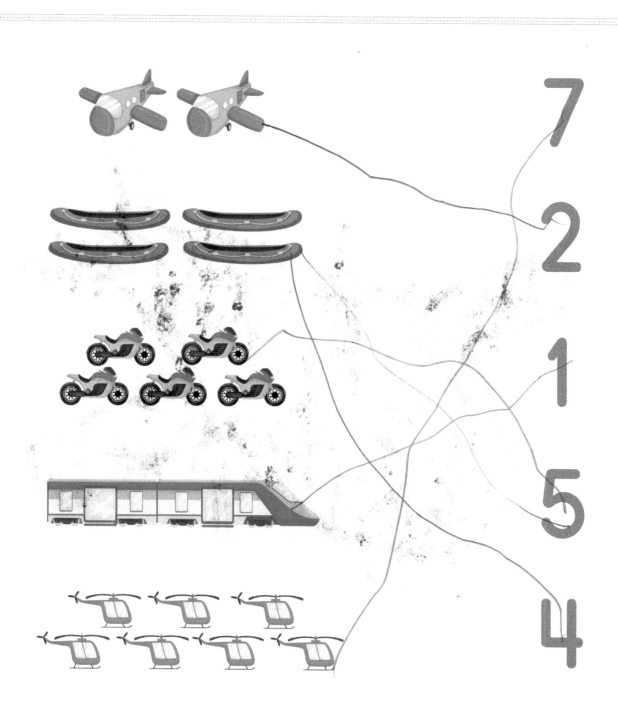

Tractor Time!

Connect the dots from 1 to 10 to complete the
tractor so it can get to work on the farm.

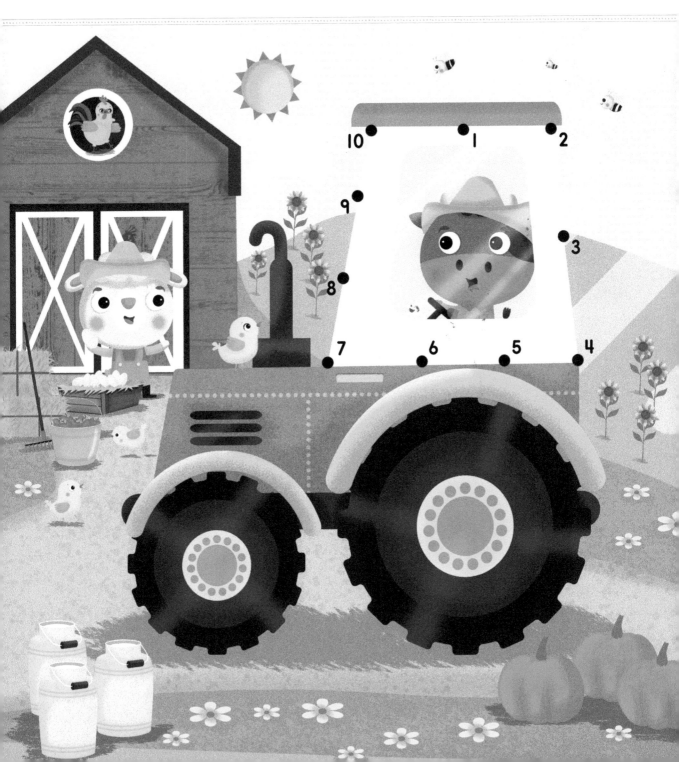

Number in the Middle

Trace the number in the middle train car in each row.

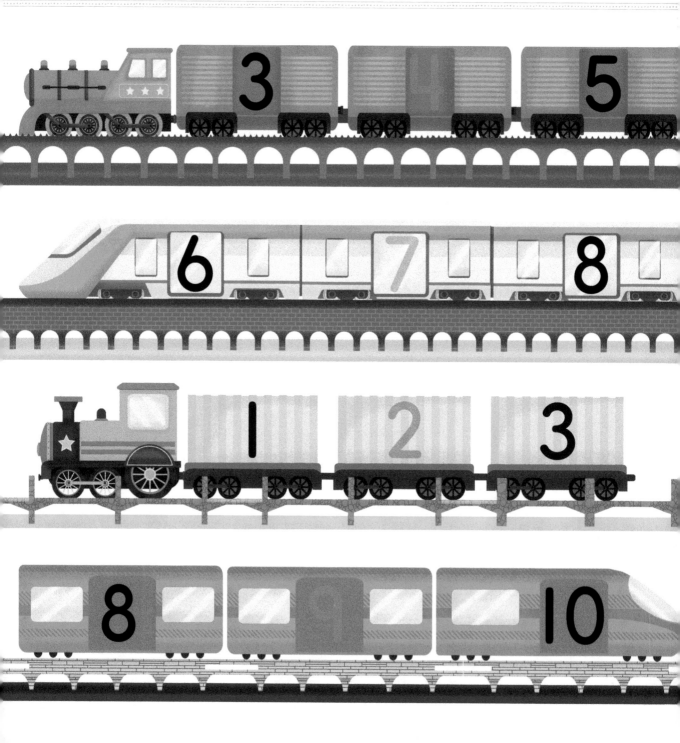

Now Boarding

Some of these airplane seats are missing numbers.
Fill in the number that comes next in each row.

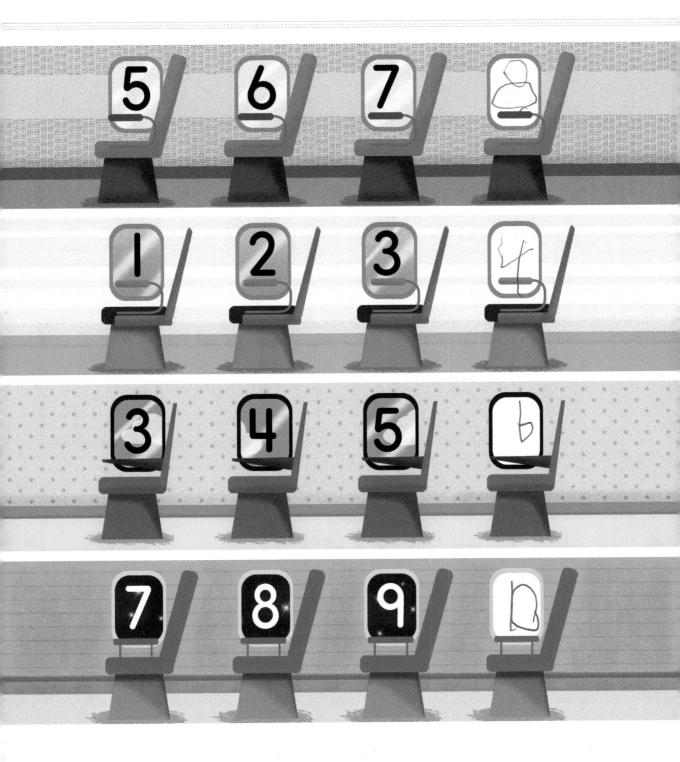

Say & Sort

This mechanic has a lot of work to do! She has to fix one
vehicle or travel word for each letter of the alphabet.
Point to and say each letter out loud.

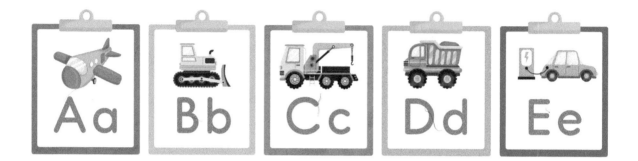

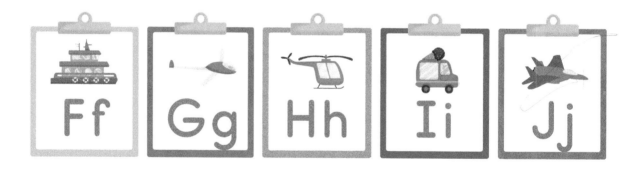

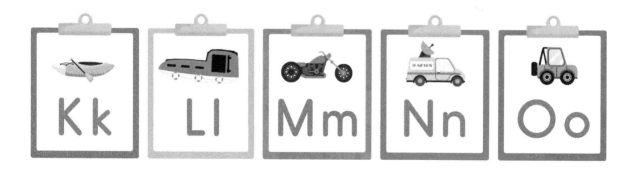

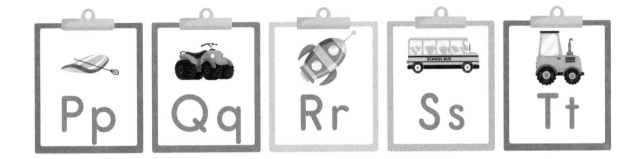

Pp Qq Rr Ss Tt

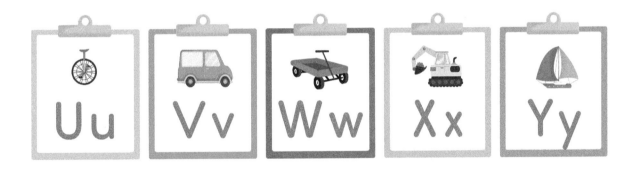

Uu Vv Ww Xx Yy

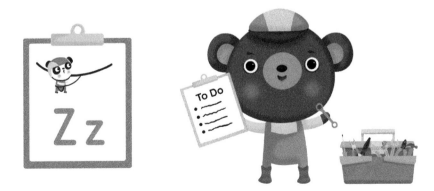

Zz

To Do

A Is for Airplane

Trace the letters and then write your own.
Connect the dots to complete the airplane so
it can fly in the sky!

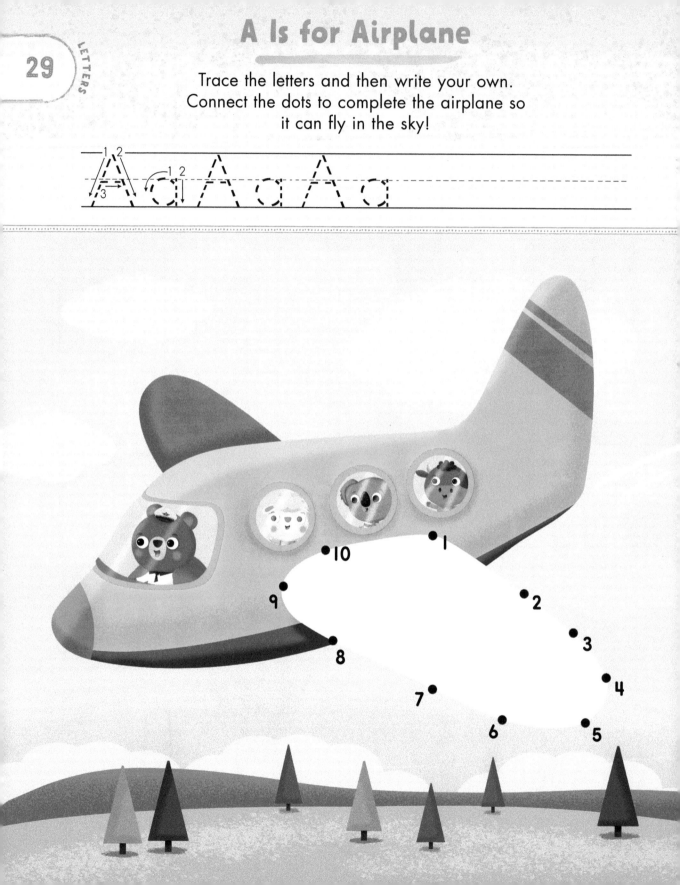

B Is for Bulldozer

Trace the letters and then write your own.
Follow the letter B to help the bulldozer
get to the construction site.

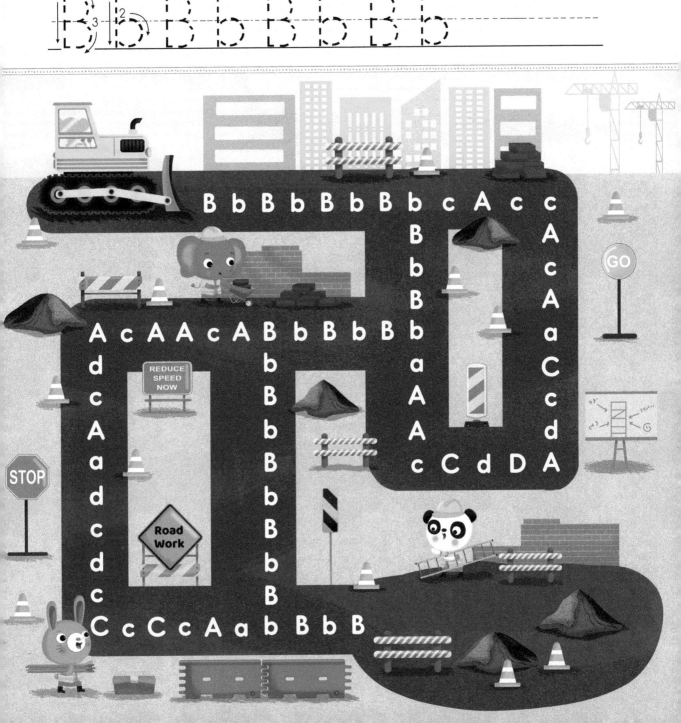

C Is for Crane

Trace and write!

Color all the spaces with the letter C yellow to make a crane.

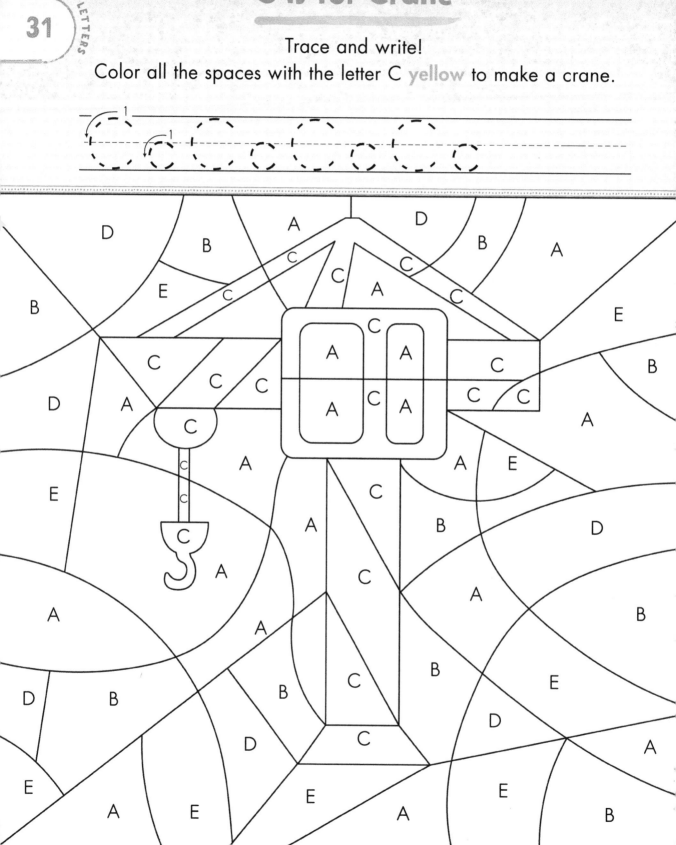

D Is for Dump Truck

Trace and write!
Match the dump truck to its pile of rocks at the quarry.

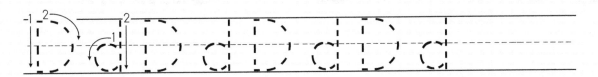

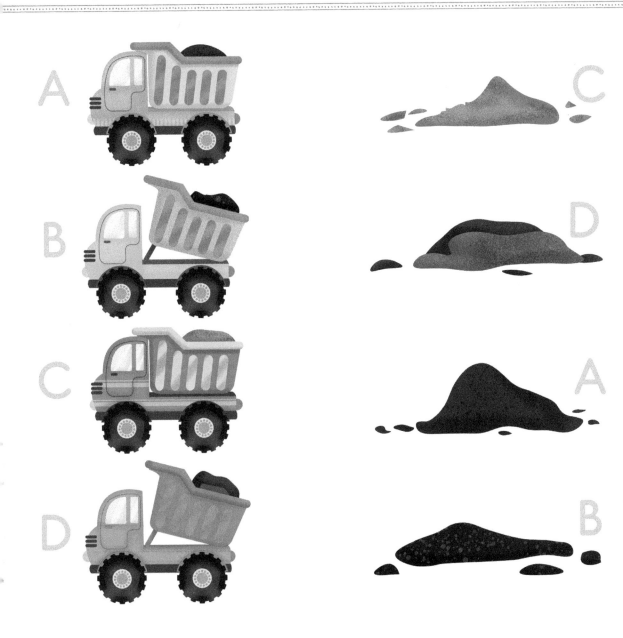

E Is for Electric Car

Trace and write!
Find and circle every letter E.

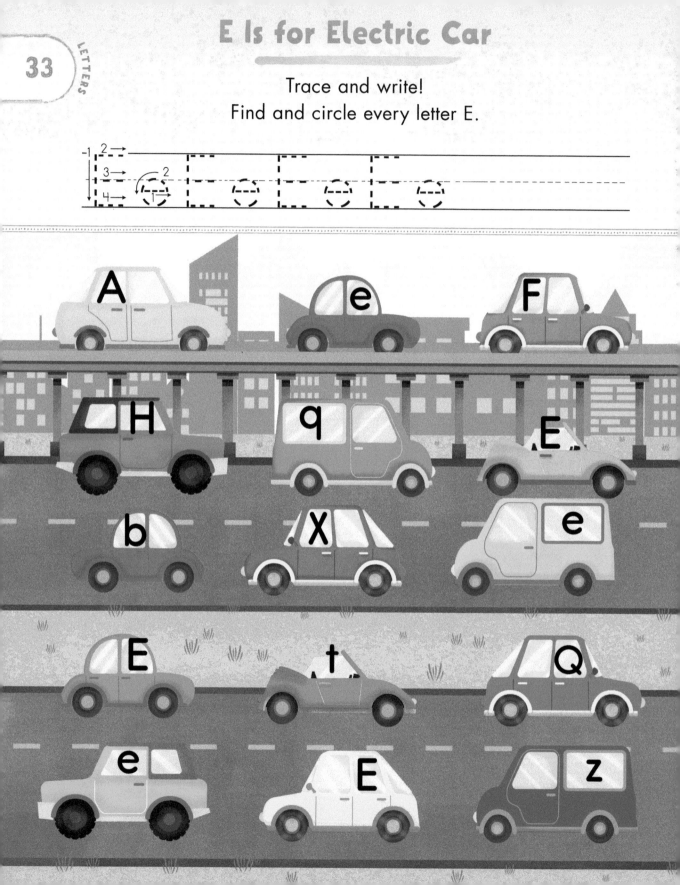

F Is for Ferry

Trace and write!
Look closely at both pictures. Find and circle 5 things
that are different in the second picture.

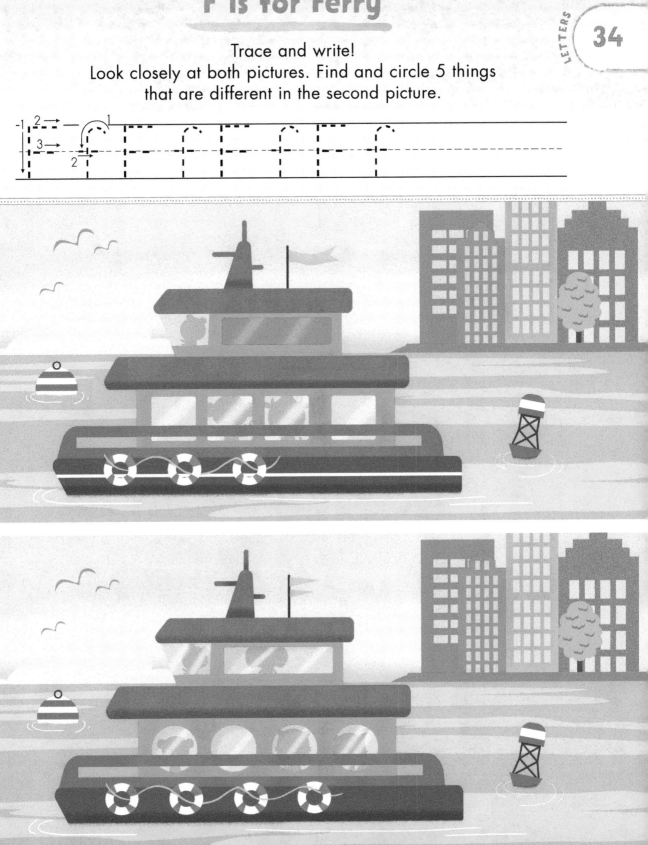

G Is for Glider

Trace and write!
Follow the letter G to fly the glider to the air show.

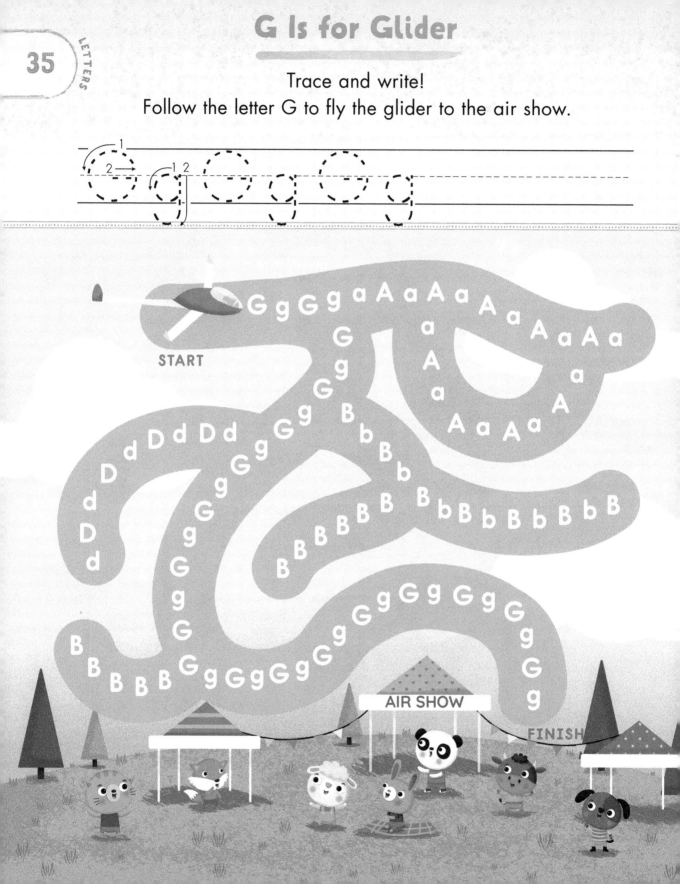

START

AIR SHOW

FINISH

H Is for Helicopter

Trace and write!
Connect the letter Hs on each blade to complete the
helicopter so it can take off!

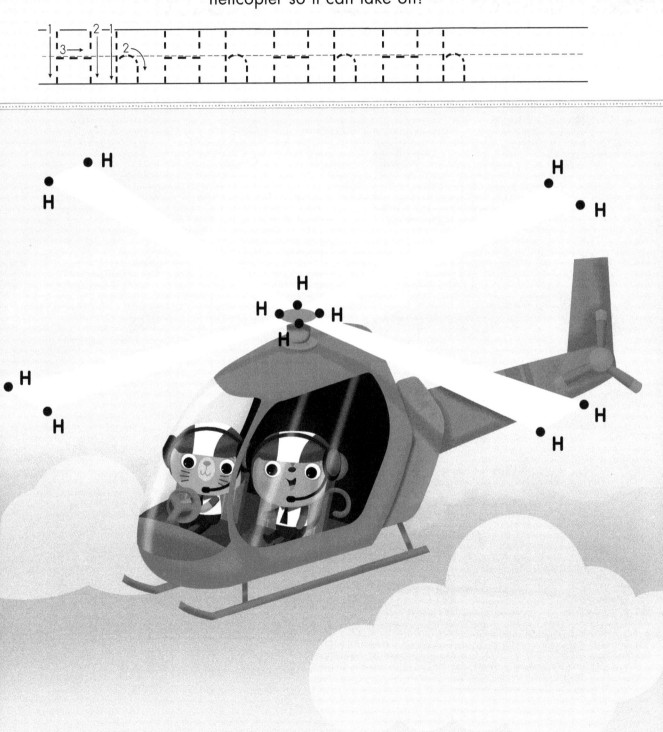

Alphabet Train

Match each train engine to the car it pulls behind it.

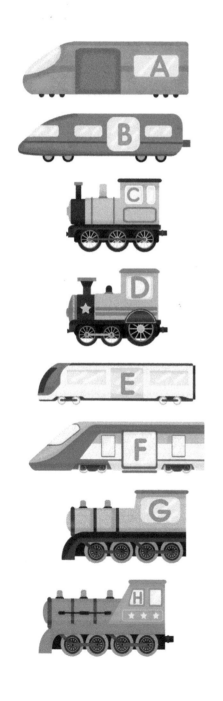

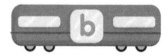

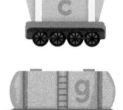

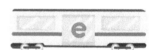

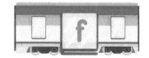

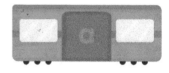

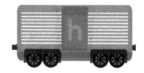

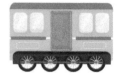

I Is for Ice Cream Truck

Trace and write!
Color the ice cream on top of the truck with your favorite flavor.
Add sprinkles that look like the letter I and i.

J Is for Jet

Trace and write!
Color all the spaces with the letter j **blue** to make a jet.

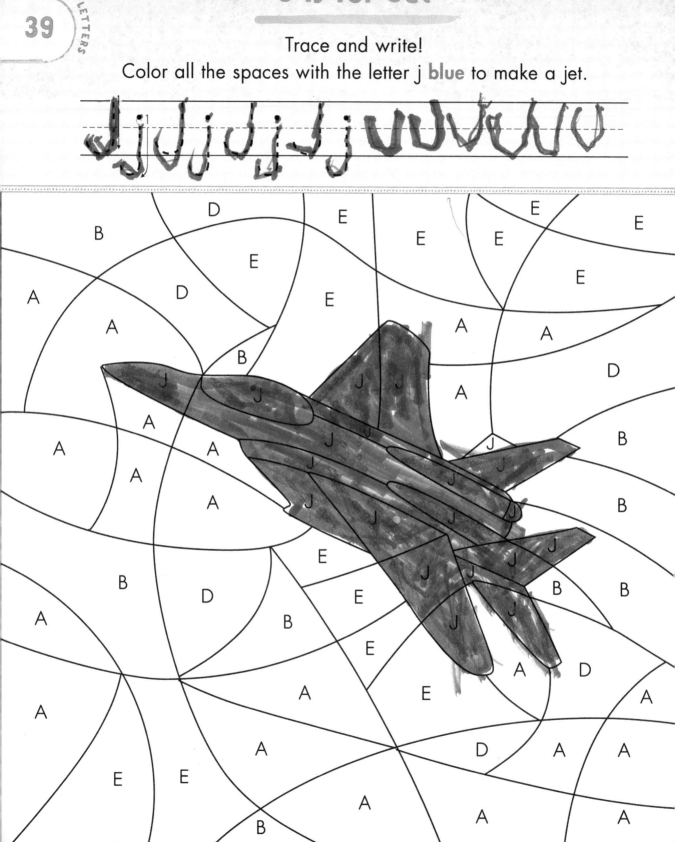

K Is for Kayak

Trace and write!
Color the kayak that comes next.

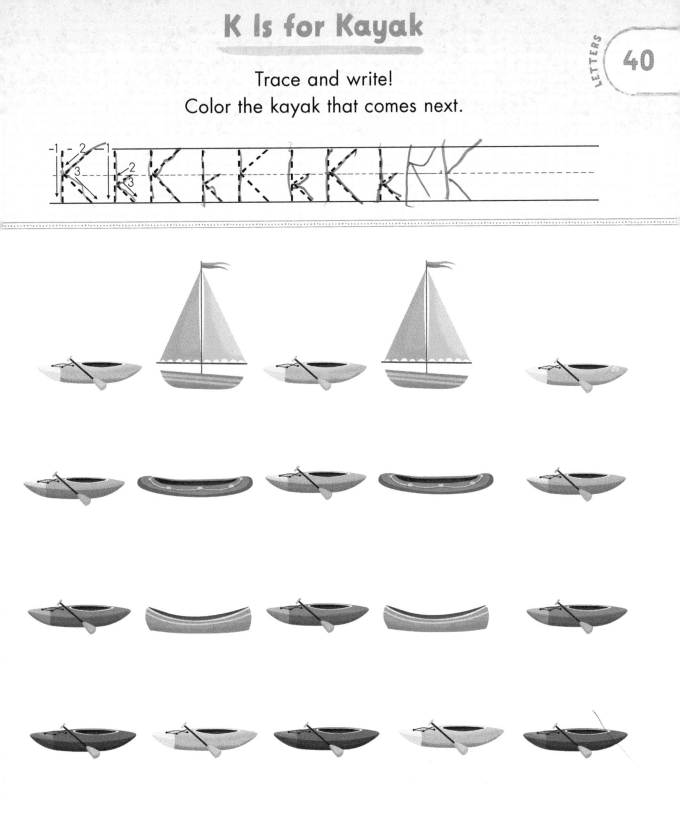

L Is for Lifeboat

Trace and write!
Draw an X on the lifeboat with the letter L.

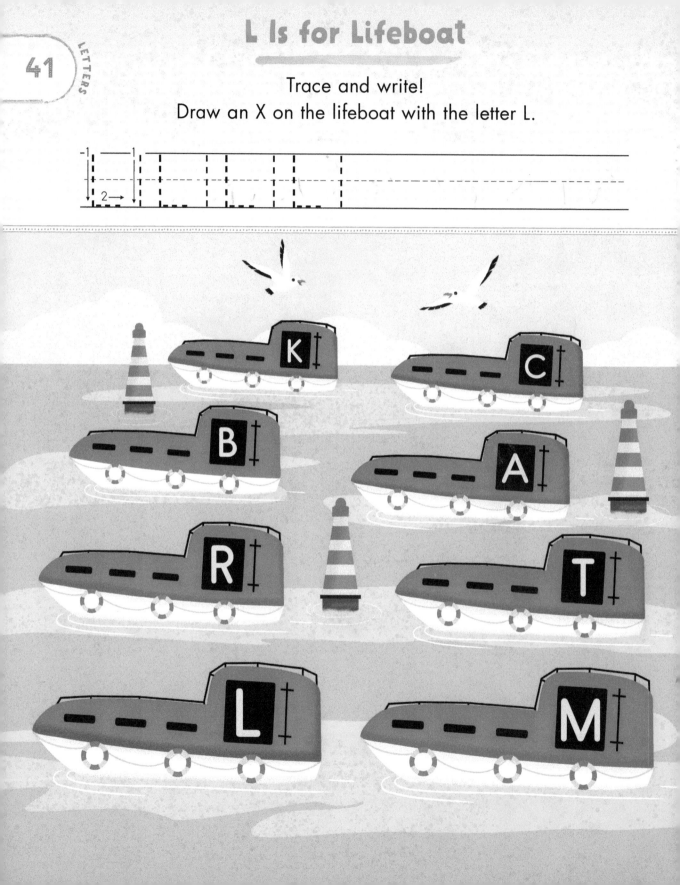

M Is for Motorcycle

Trace and write!
Draw a line from the motorcycle to its shadow.

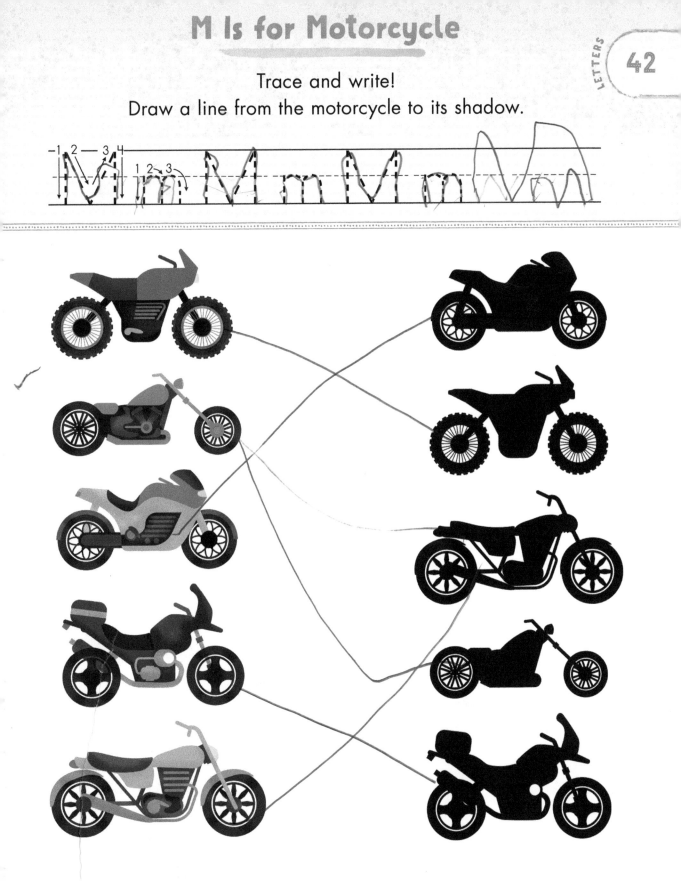

N Is for News Van

Trace and write!
Connect the dots from A to N to make the satellite dish
for this news van so it can broadcast the news!

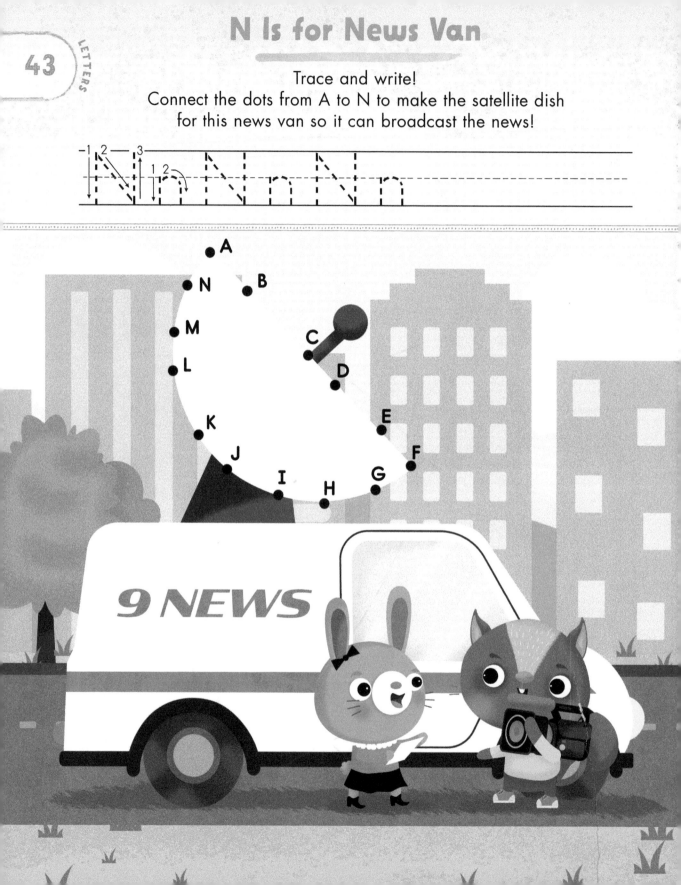

O Is for Off-Road Vehicle

Trace and write!
Follow the letter O to help the off-road
vehicle get to the campsite.

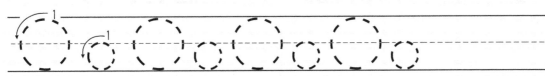

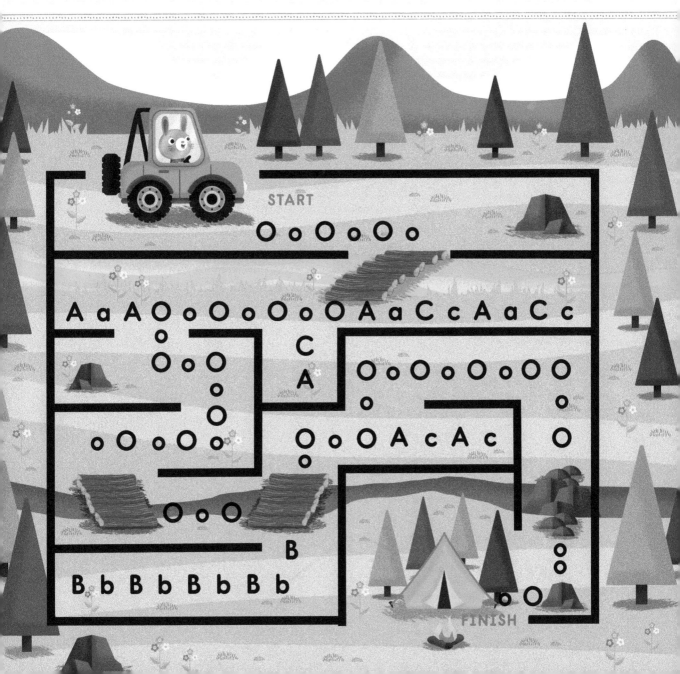

P Is for Paddleboard

Trace and write!
Color the paddleboards **blue** and **red**.

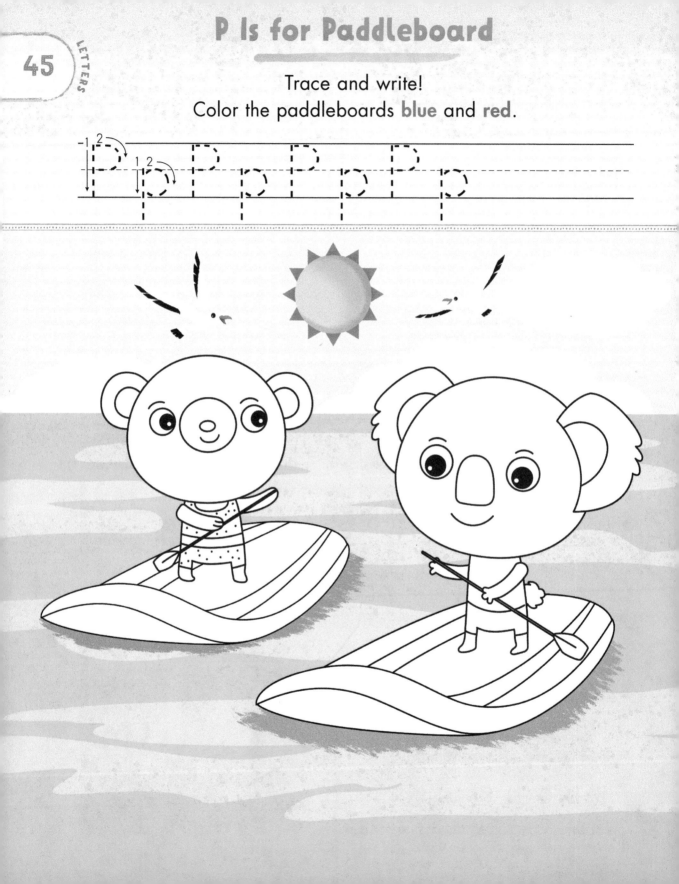

Q Is for Quad Bike

Trace and write!
Circle the tire that matches its quad bike.

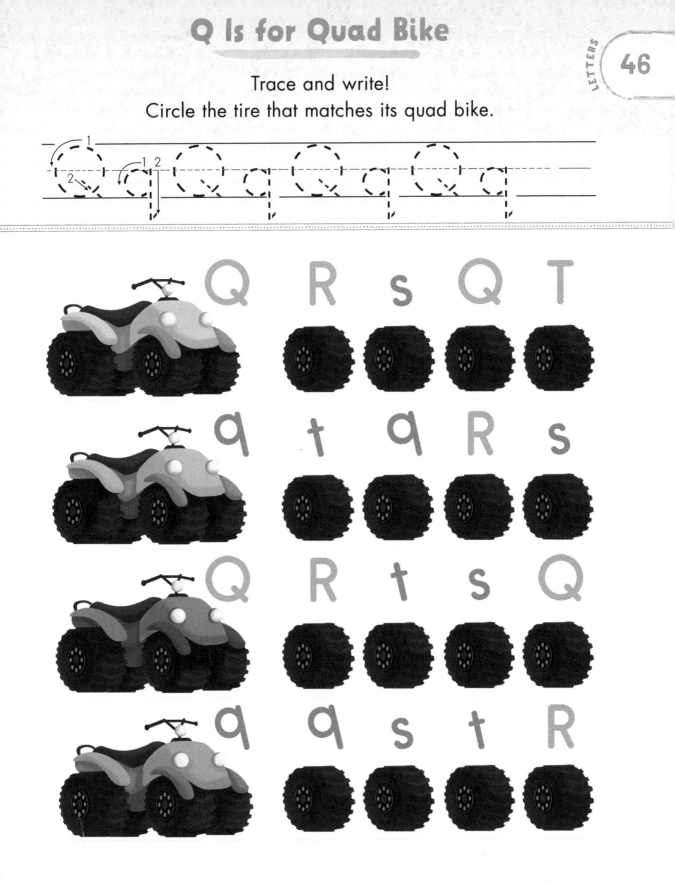

Q   R   s   Q   T

q   t   q   R   s

Q   R   t   s   Q

q   q   s   t   R

Just Plane Awesome

Trace the letters I J K L M N O P Q in the sky!

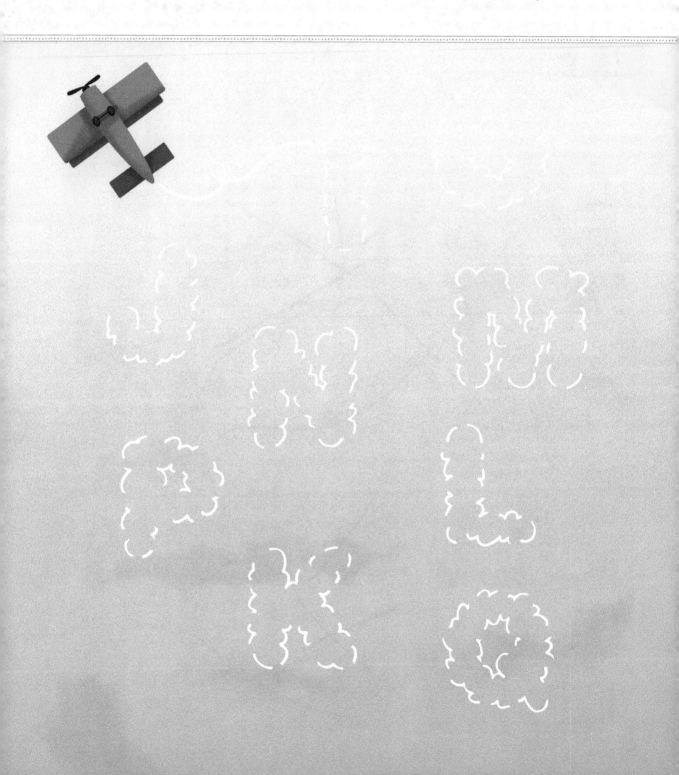

R Is for Rocket

Trace and write!
Circle all of the rockets with the letter R.

R R r R r R r R r

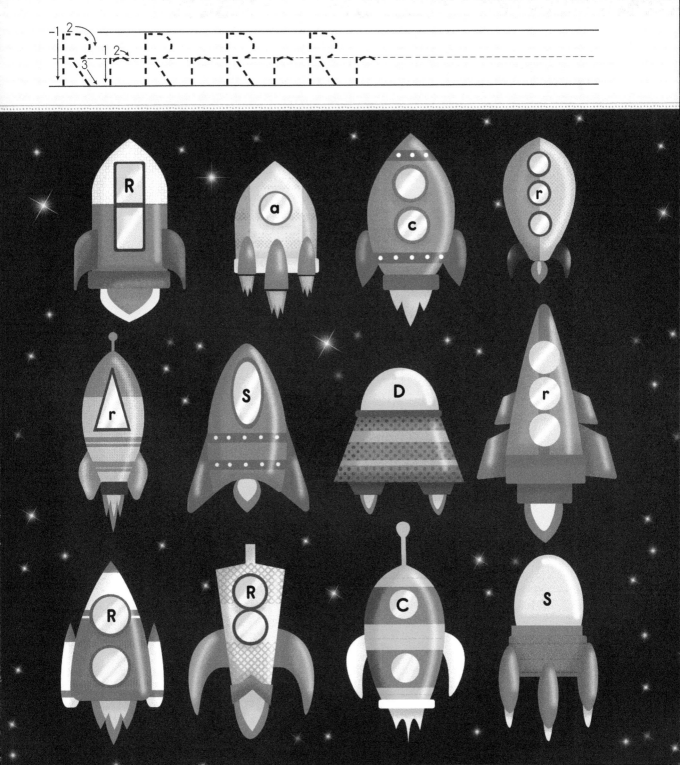

S Is for School Bus

Trace and write!
Trace the missing letter.

S s S s S s S s

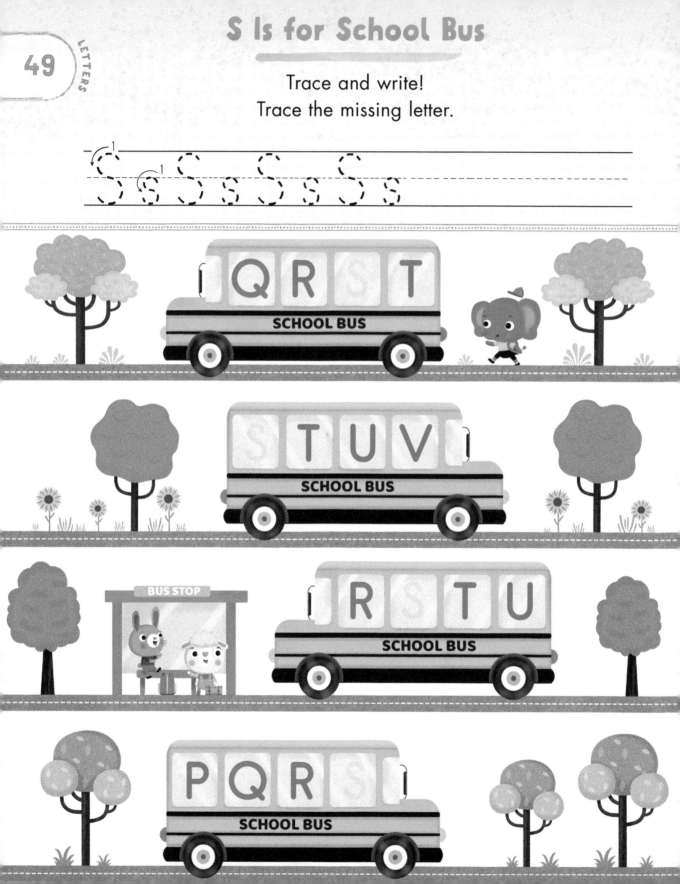

Q R S T
SCHOOL BUS

S T U V
SCHOOL BUS

R S T U
BUS STOP
SCHOOL BUS

P Q R S
SCHOOL BUS

T Is for Tractor

Trace and write!
Help the tractor follow the letter T to get to the barn.

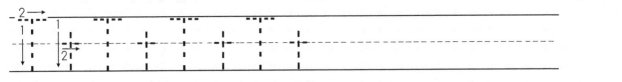

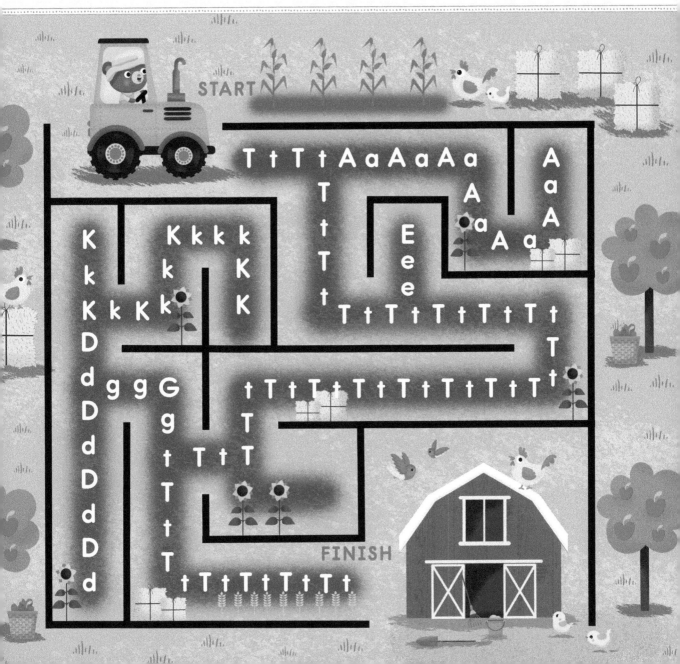

U Is for Unicycle

Trace and write!
Connect the dots from A to U to make
this unicycle extra sturdy!

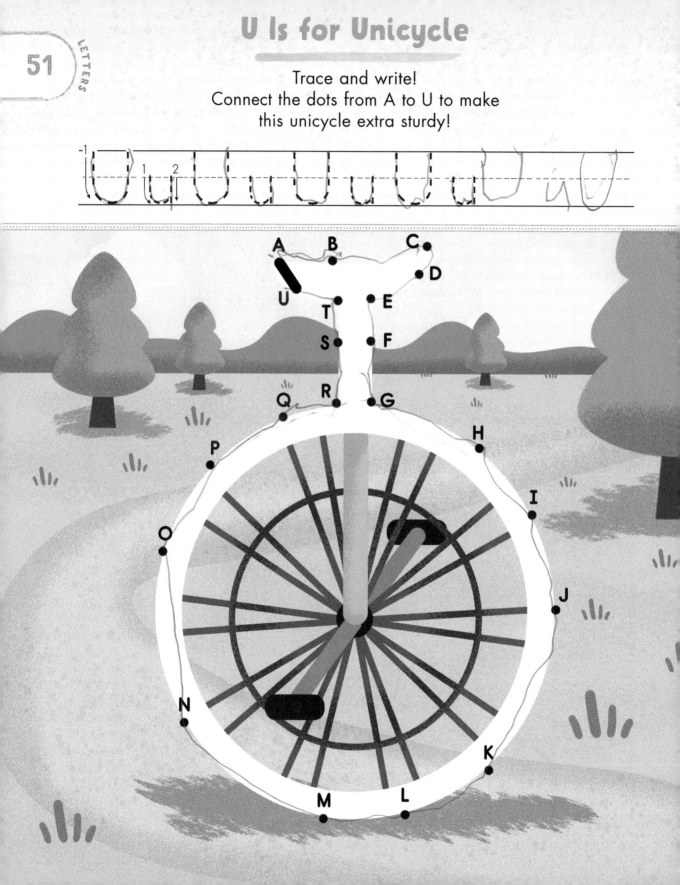

V Is for Van

Trace and write!
This van needs a new paint job! Color the van **purple**.

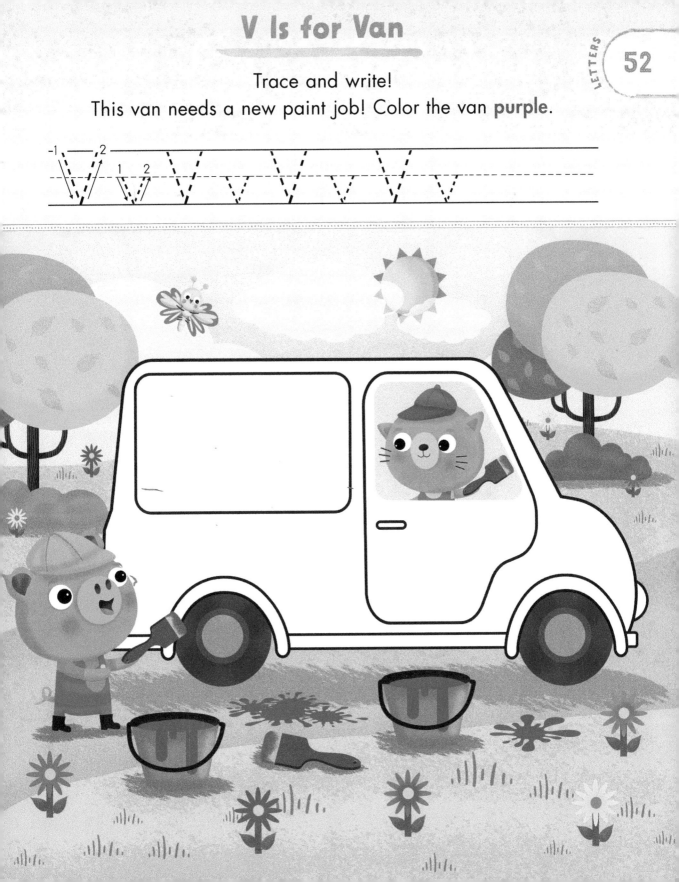

W Is for Wagon

Trace and write!
Find and circle the 2 wagons that are exactly the same.

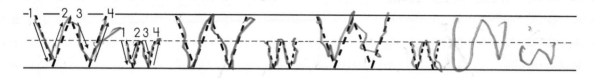

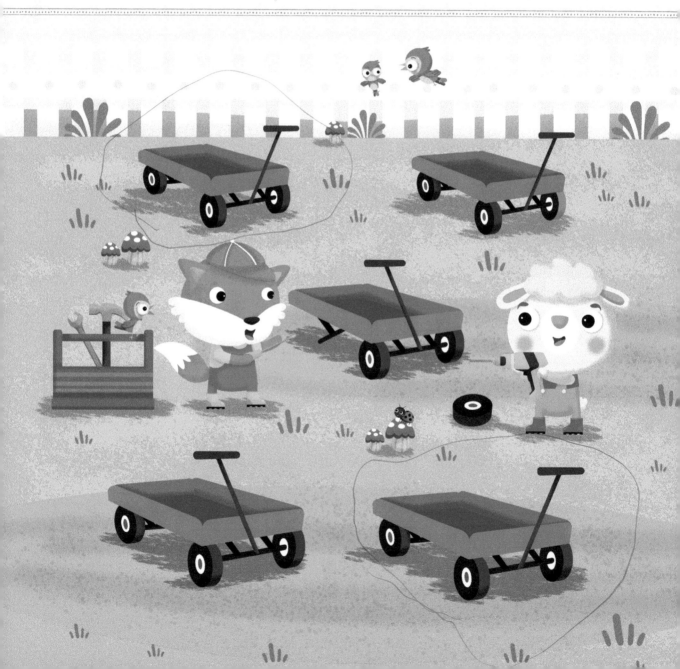

X Is in Excavator

Trace and write!
This excavator needs to know where to dig.
Circle all the digging sites marked with an X.

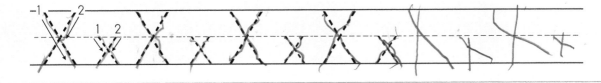

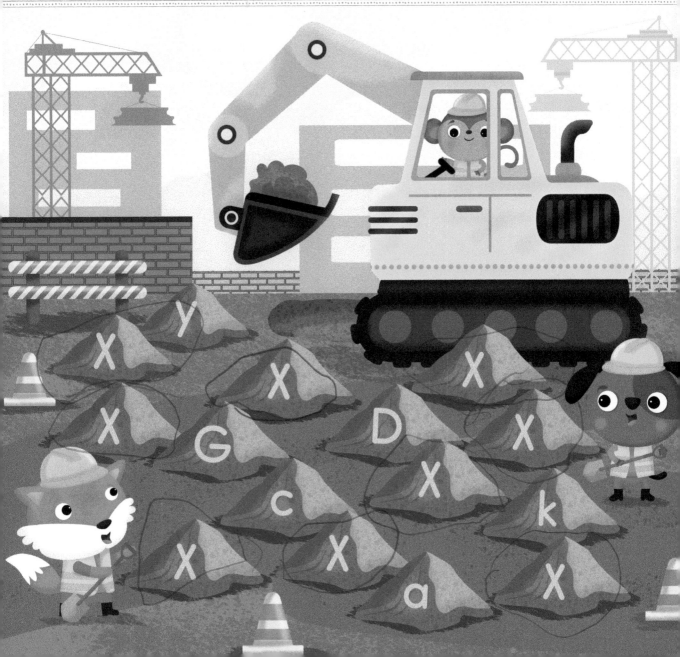

Y Is for Yacht

Trace and write!
Draw a line to match the front of each yacht to its back.

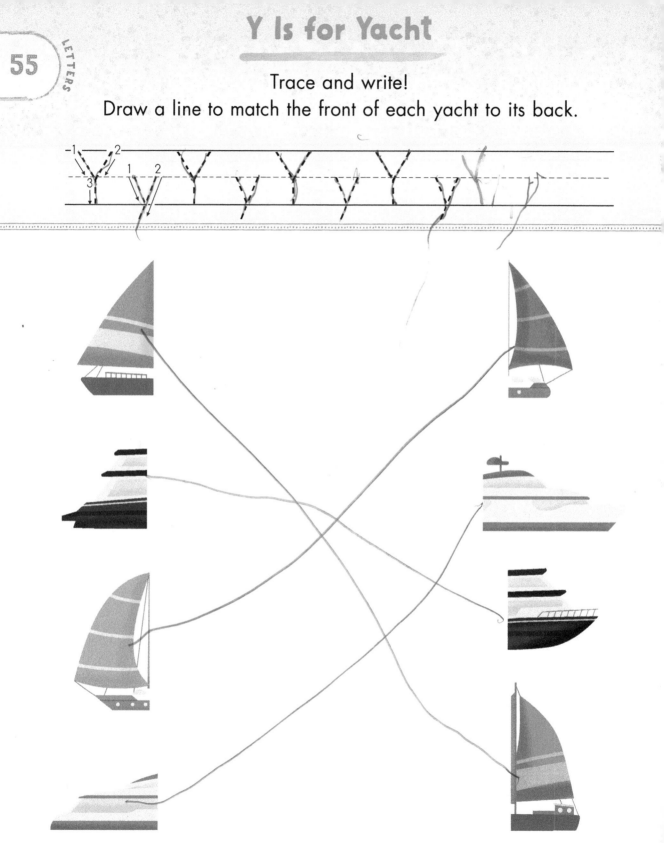

Z Is for Zip Line

Trace and write!
Follow the letter Z to help this zip line
rider through the treetop maze.

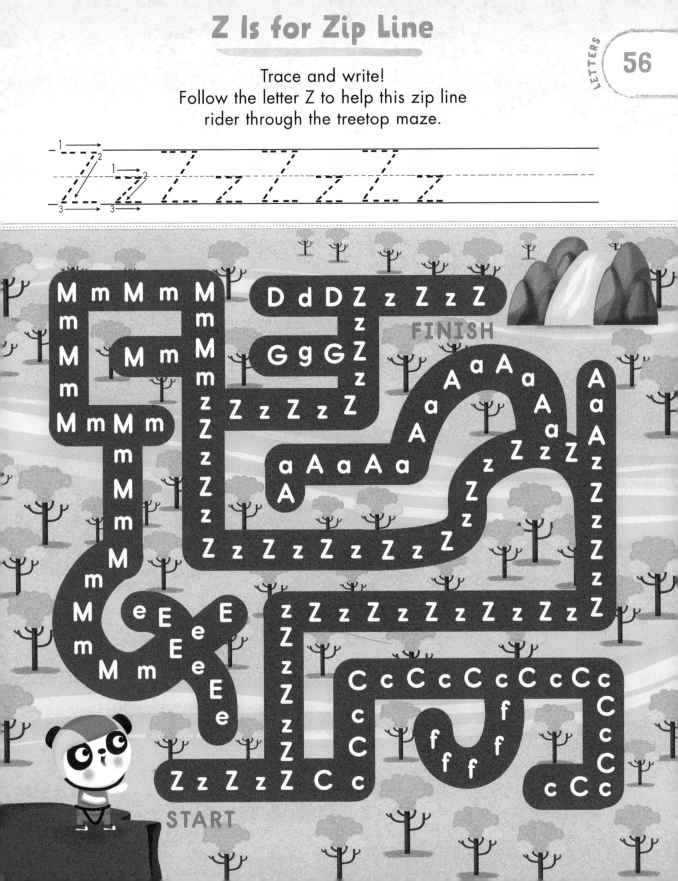

All Under Control

Connect the dots from A to Z so this airport's control tower can be ready to guide airplanes coming and going!

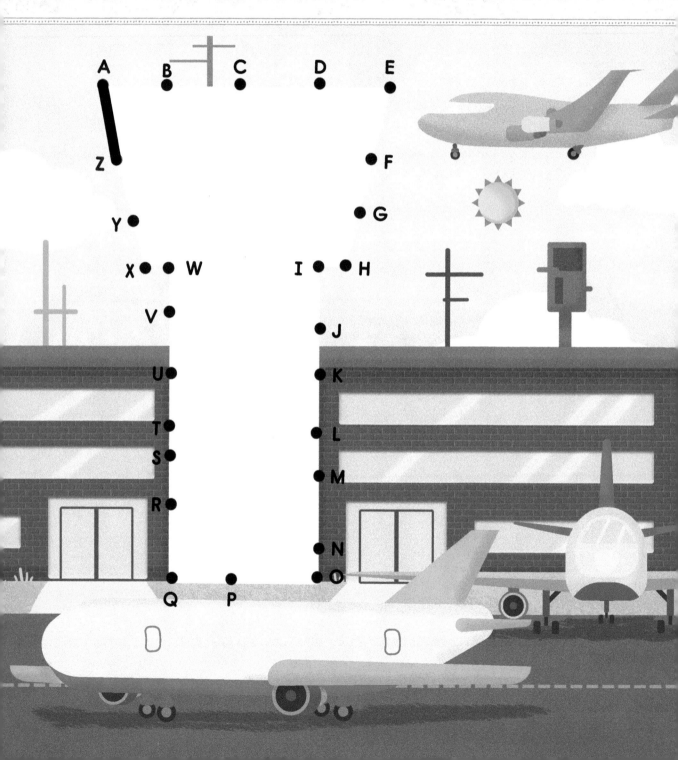

Blast Off!

Follow the alphabet from A to Z to help the rocket get to the moon as quickly as you can. Try singing the ABC song at the same time!

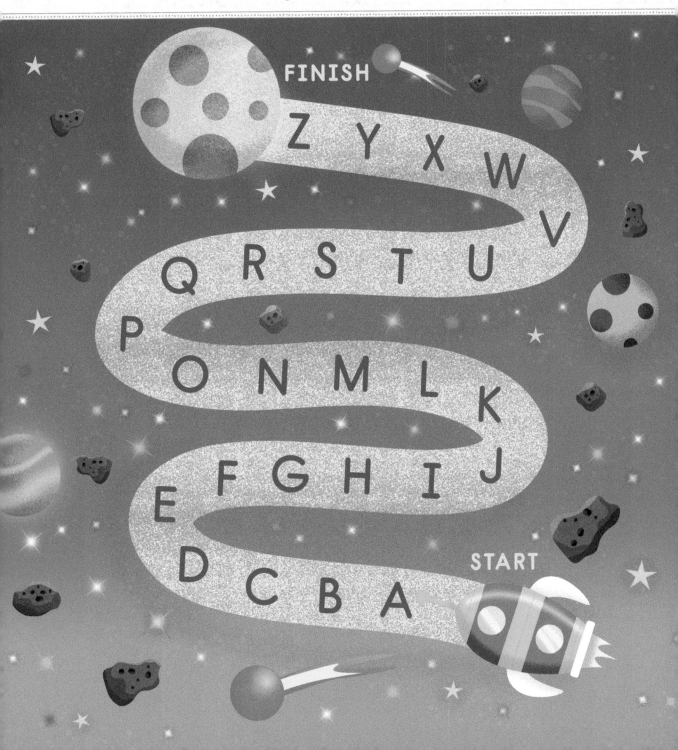

Showtime!

Trace the word as quickly as you can
so the car can get going!
Take each of these cars for a spin by tracing the lines.

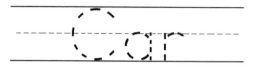

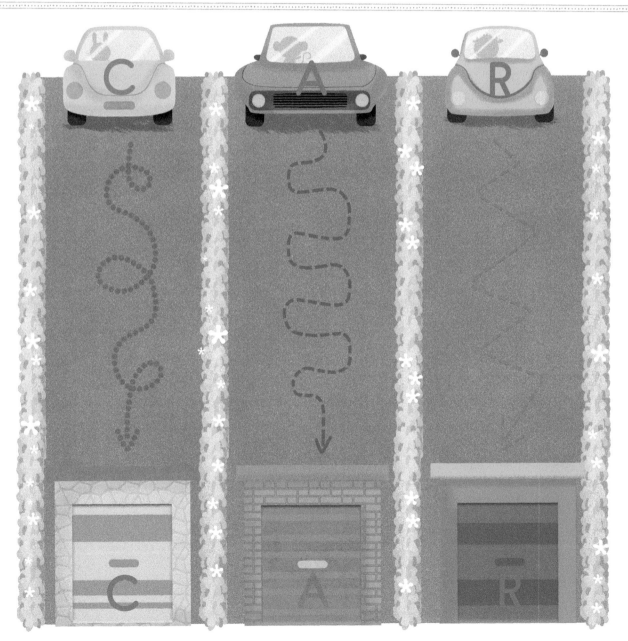

Flying Fun

Trace the word so the jet can soar!
Look closely at both pictures. Find and circle
4 differences in the second picture.

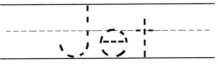

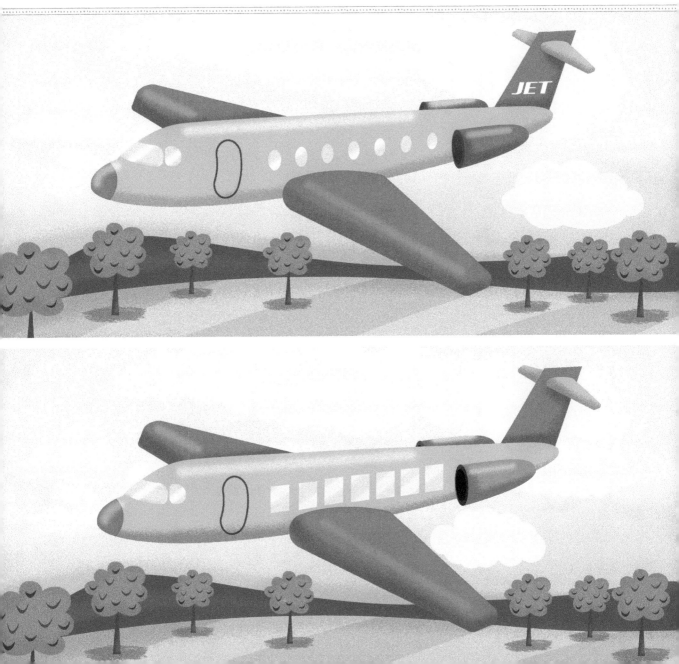

Busy Boats

Trace the word for some smooth sailing!
Find and circle each of the words in the puzzle below.
Be sure to look up, down, left, and right.

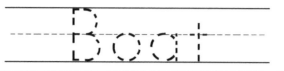

Boat

BOAT   **SHIP**

OAR   **SEA**

DOCK   **WAVE**

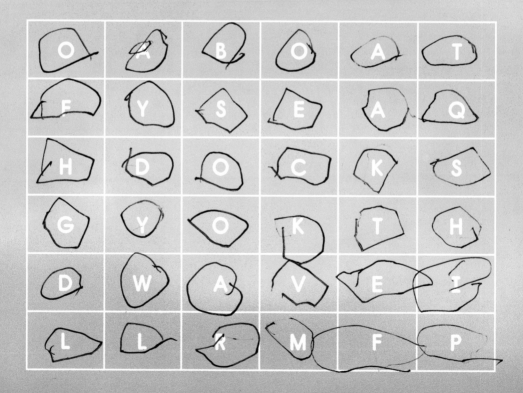

O	A	B	O	A	T
F	Y	S	E	A	Q
H	D	O	C	K	S
G	Y	O	K	T	H
D	W	A	V	E	I
L	L	R	M	F	P

The Beginning Letter

Say each vehicle's name out loud and circle its first letter.

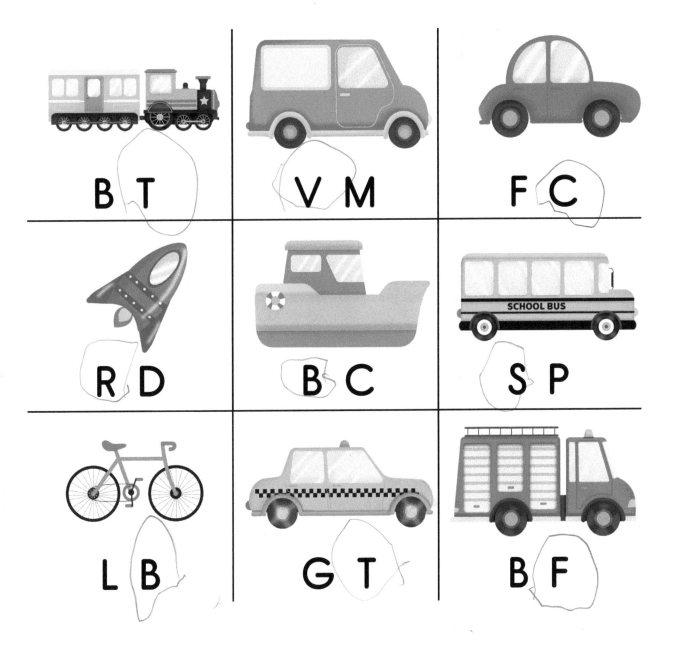

B T

V M

F C

R D

B C

S P

L B

G T

B F

The Right Name

Match each vehicle to its name.

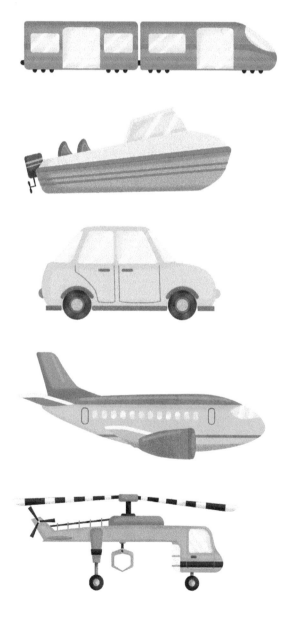

AIRPLANE

HELICOPTER

TRAIN

BOAT

CAR

The Missing Letter

Fill in the blank to complete each word.

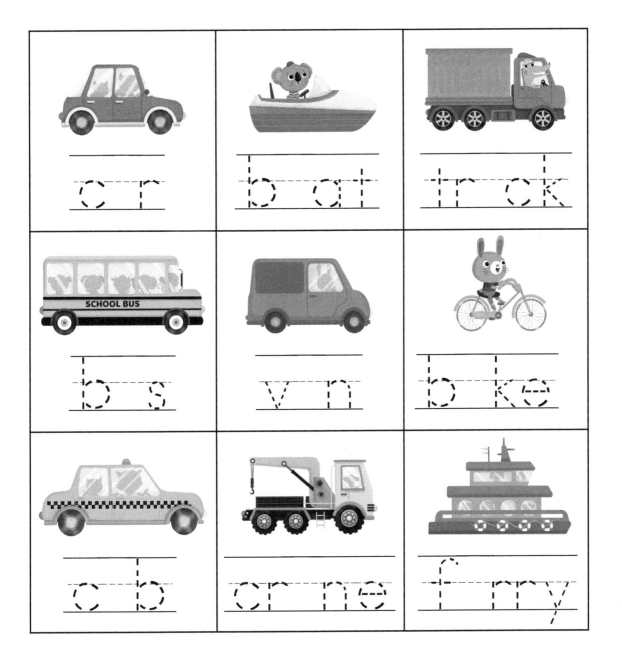

c _ r

b o a t

t r _ c k

b _ s

v _ n

b _ ke

c _ b

cr _ ne

f _ rry

Wheely Fast!

Trace the circles. Can you see how round they are?
Color the tires to give this race car new wheels.

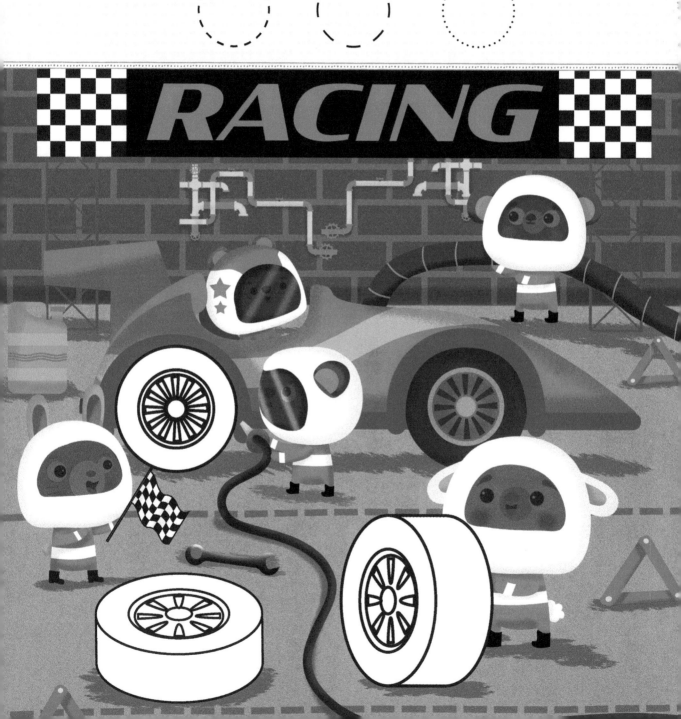

Fair & Square

Trace the squares.
Find and color all the squares in the picture below.

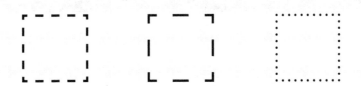

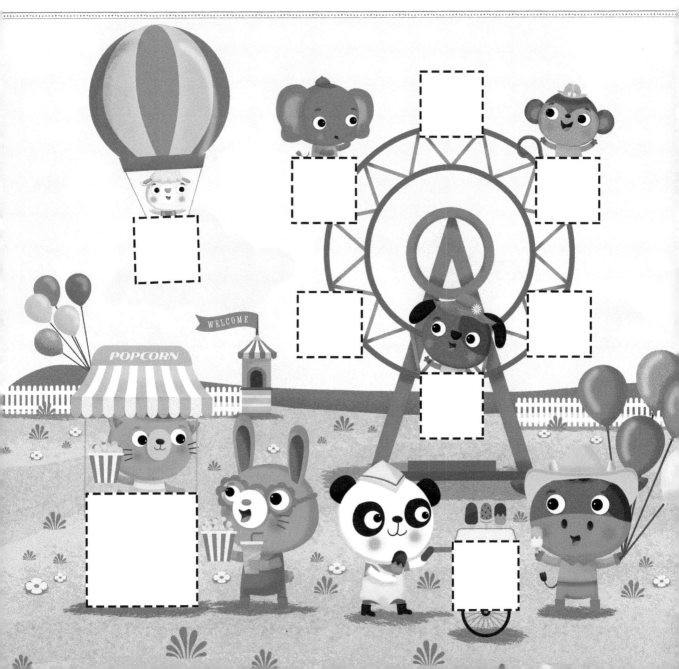

Follow the Rectangles

Trace the rectangles.
Follow the rectangles to help the fire truck
get back to the station.

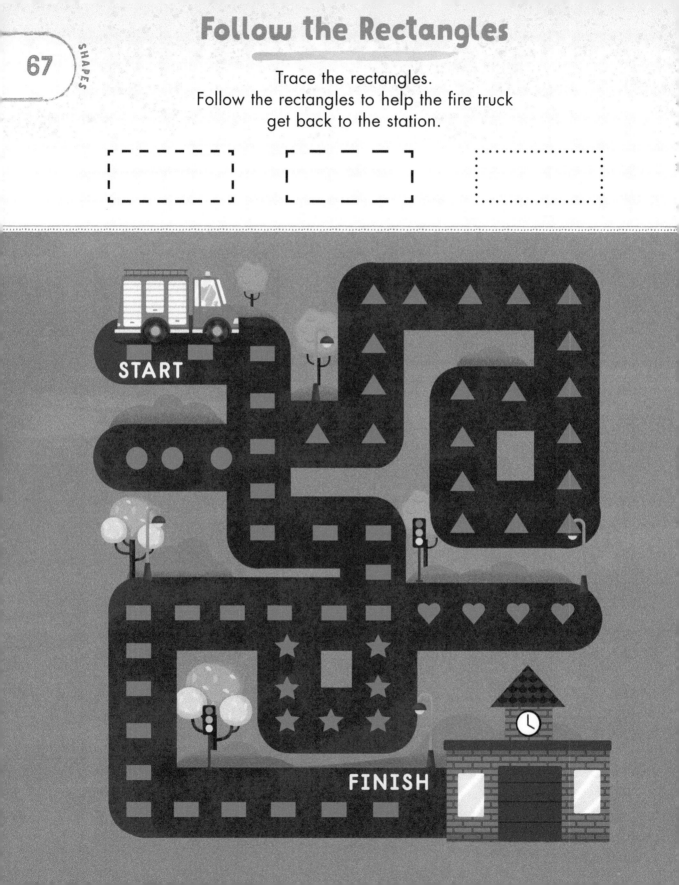

Triangle Time!

Trace the triangles.
Draw an X on all 7 triangles you see in the picture below.

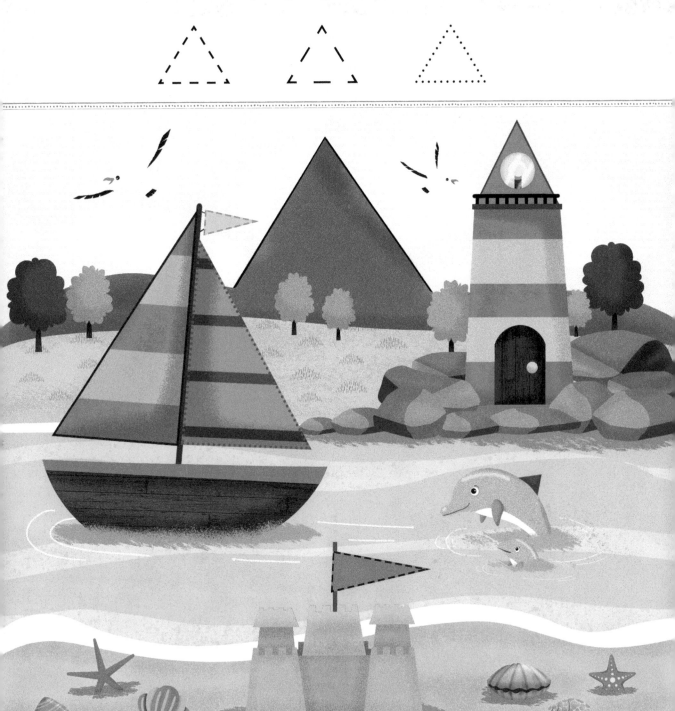

All Mixed Up

Trace the ovals.
Connect the dots so this truck can start mixing concrete!

Digging for Diamonds

Trace the diamonds.
Circle the shape that completes the pattern.

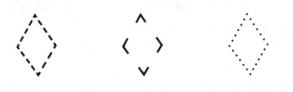

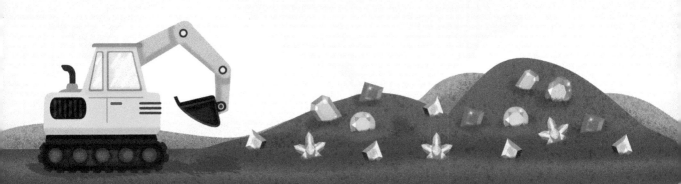

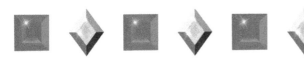

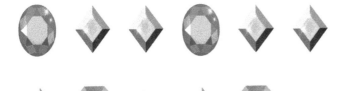

Lost Love Letters

Trace the hearts.
This mail truck is filled with valentines! Draw lines to connect the
valentines for the truck.

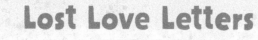

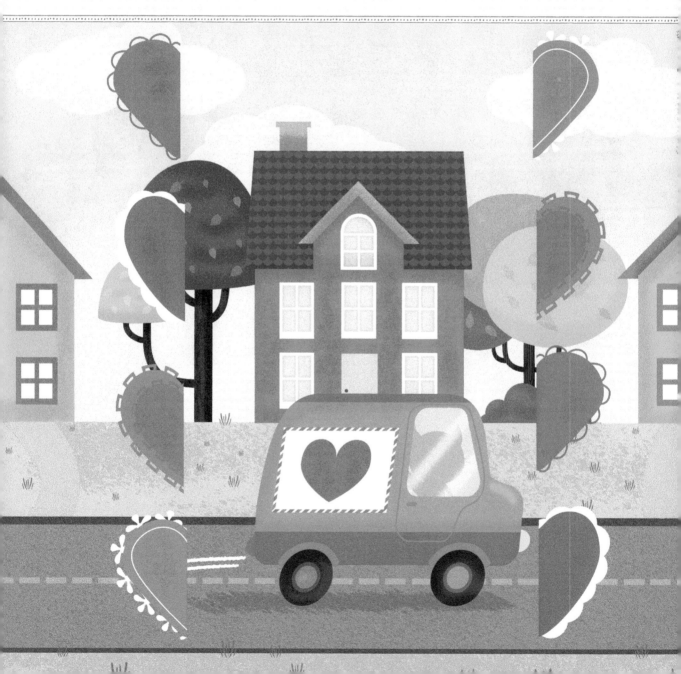

By My Stars!

Trace the stars.
Color every section with a star **blue**. What do you see?

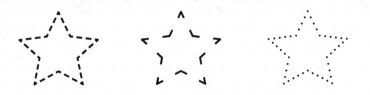

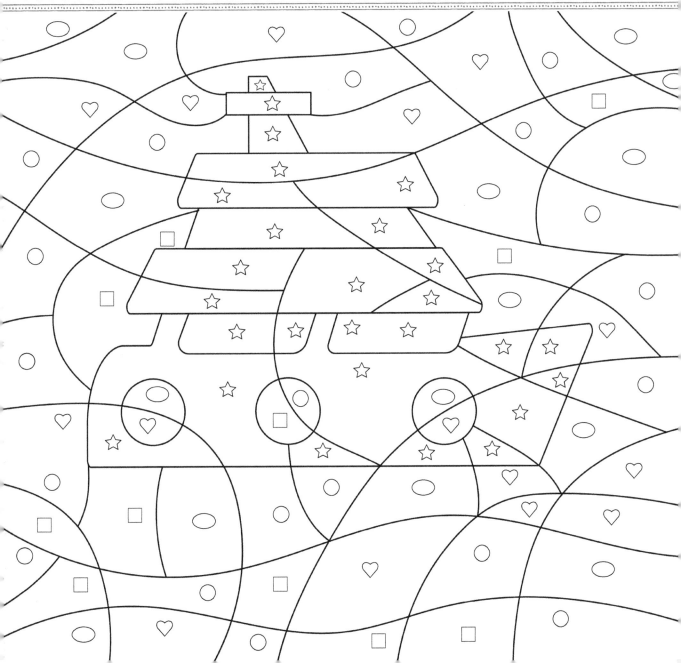

Sign Shadows

Match each road sign to its shadow.

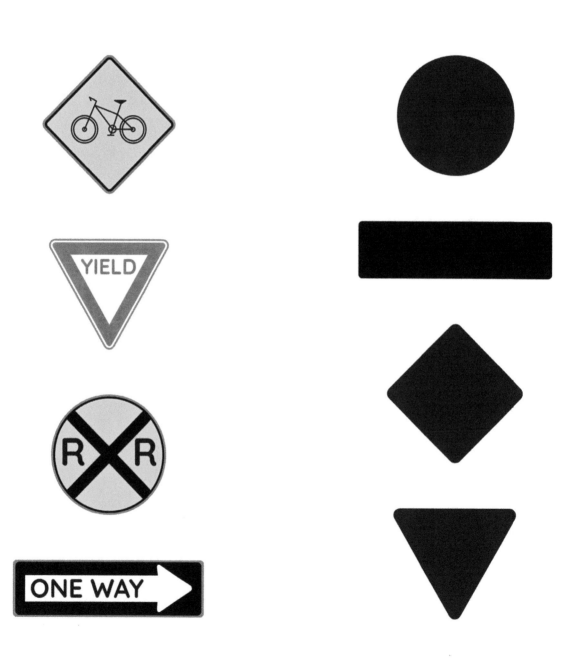

The Construction Site Takes Shape

Use the color key below to color the construction site.

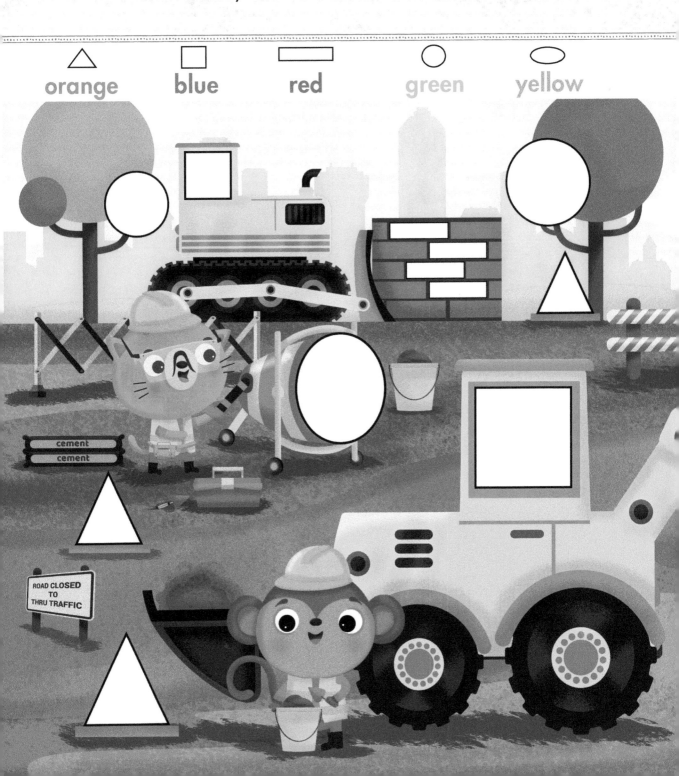

orange   blue   red   green   yellow

cement
cement

ROAD CLOSED
TO
THRU TRAFFIC

Paint Job Patterns

Match each vehicle with the close-up of its pattern.

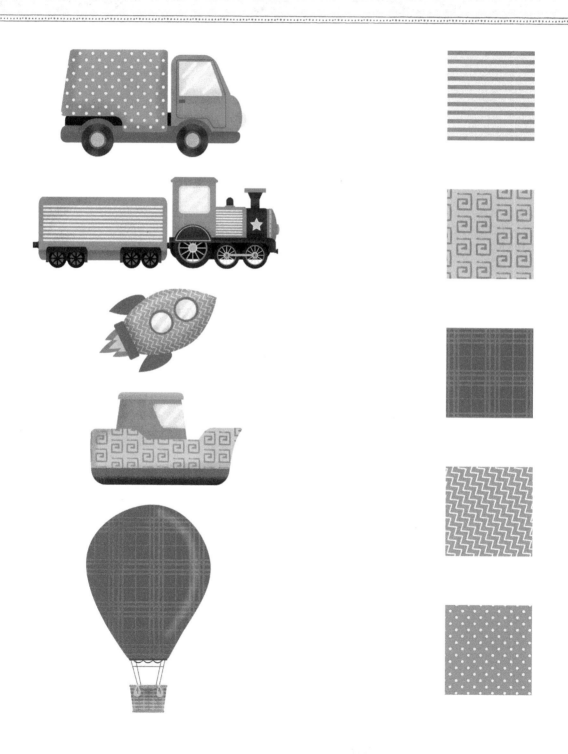

Right on Track

Color the train cars that come next.

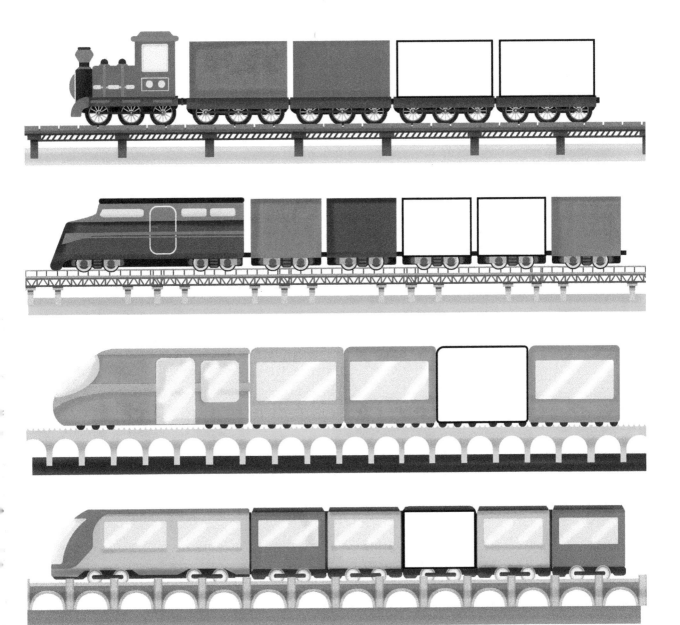

Crazy Campers

Look closely at both pictures. Find and circle 9 differences in the second picture.

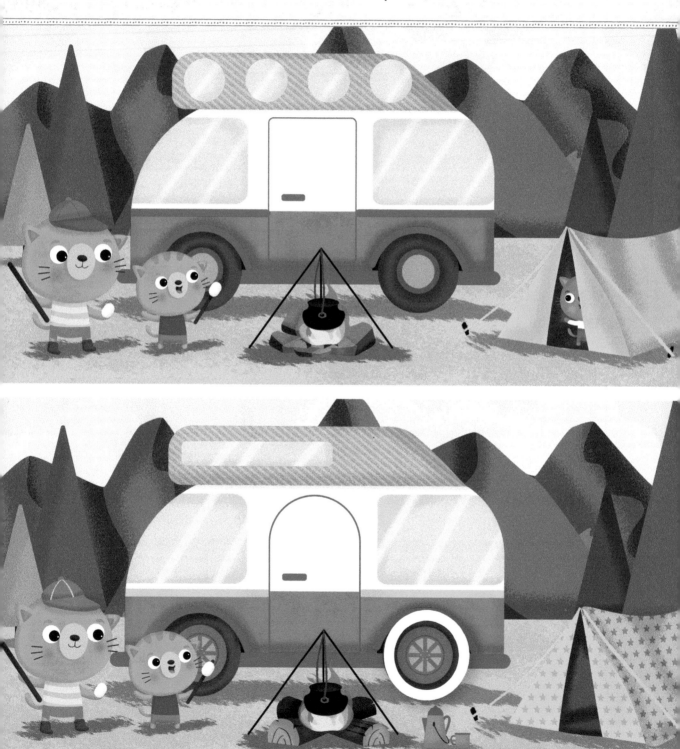

A Moving Experience

Follow this pattern to help the moving truck find its new home:

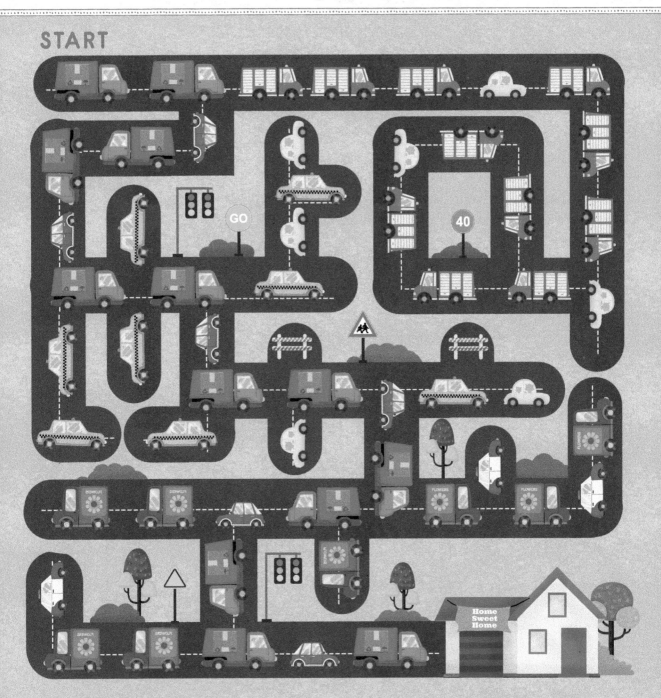

START

GO

40

Home Sweet Home

FINISH

Pattern Parade

Circle the vehicle that comes next in the parade.

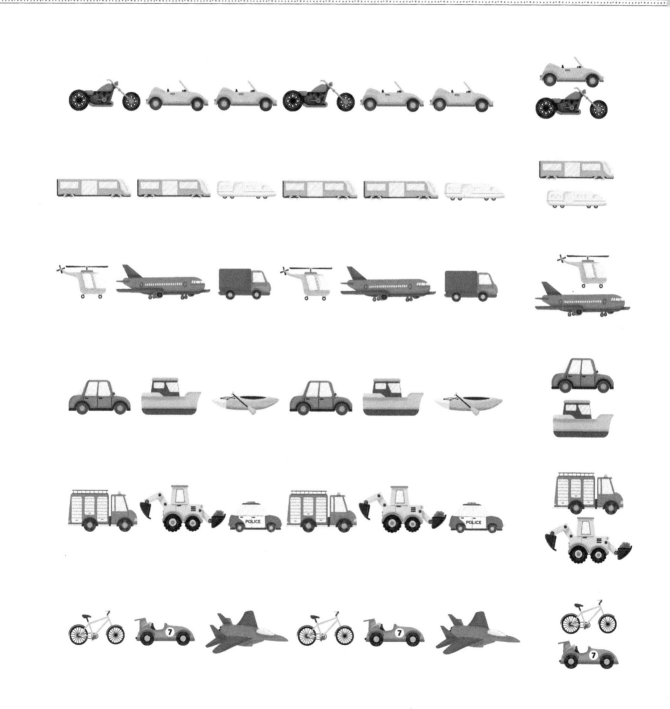

Bonkers for Bumper Cars

Color the bumper cars by their patterns.

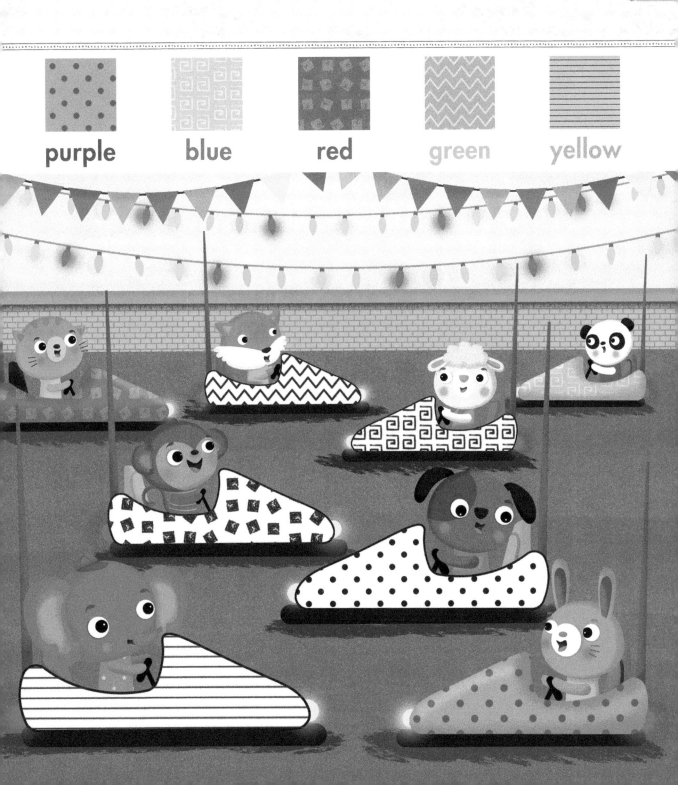

purple   **blue**   **red**   green   yellow

ANSWER KEY

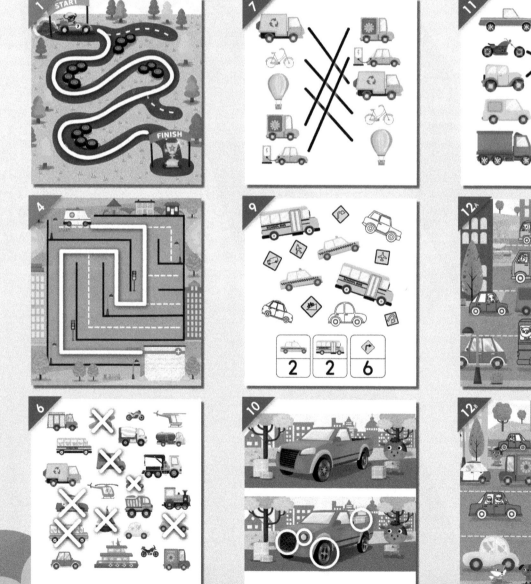
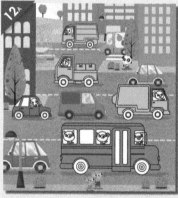
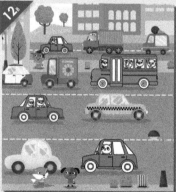

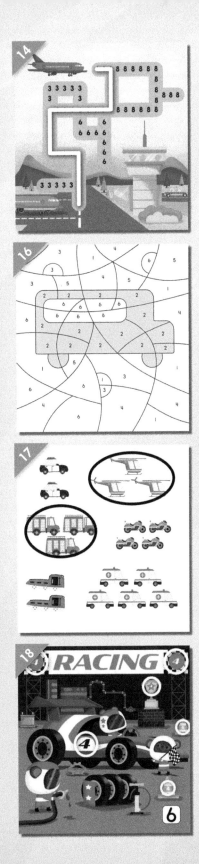

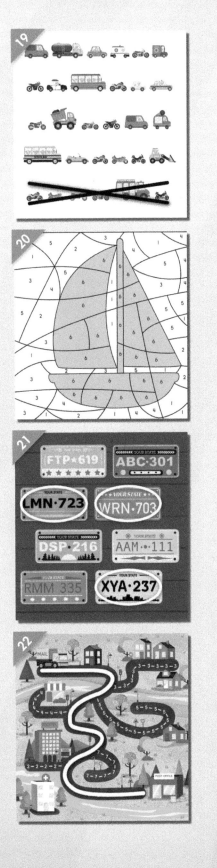

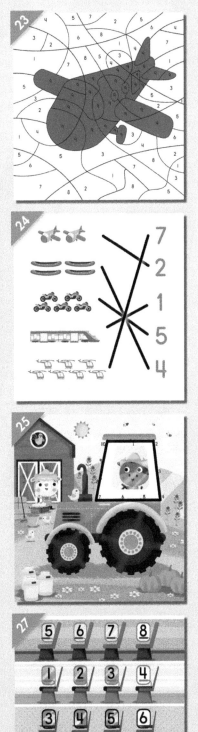

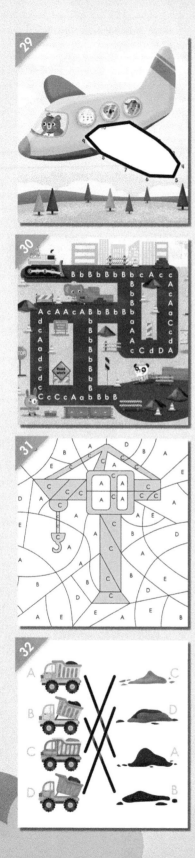

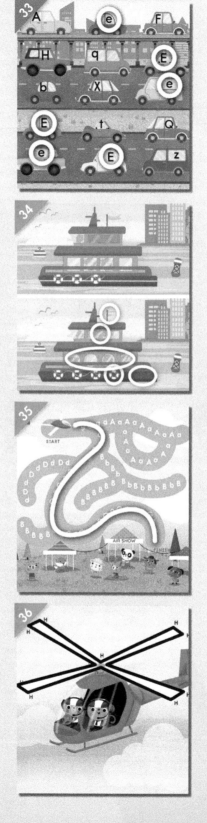

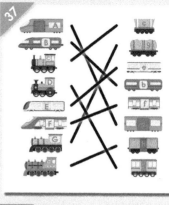

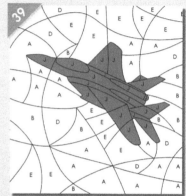

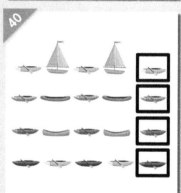

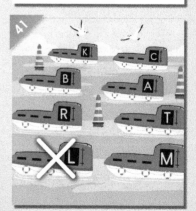

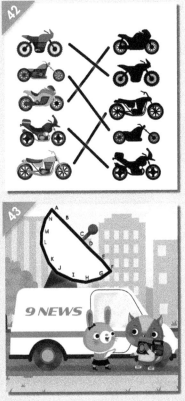

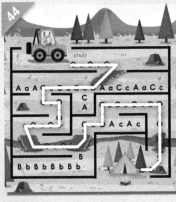

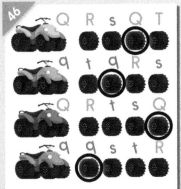

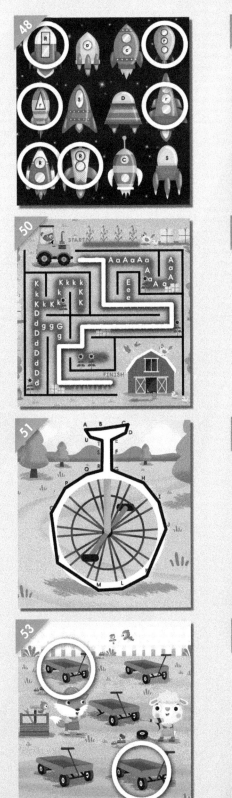

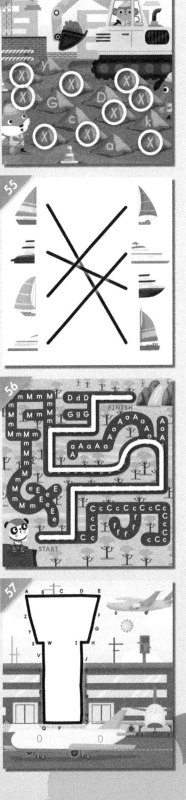

60

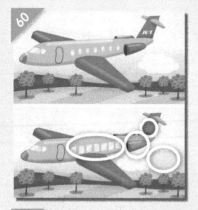

64

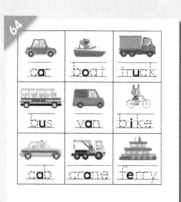

car · boat · truck
bus · van · bike
cab · crane · ferry

70

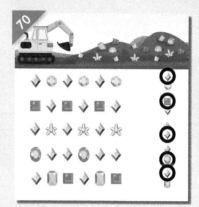

61

BOAT · SHIP
OAR · SEA
DOCK · WAVE

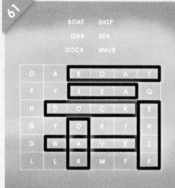

67

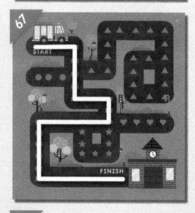

71

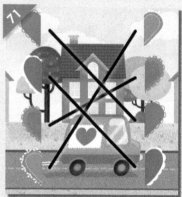

62

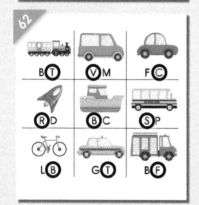

68

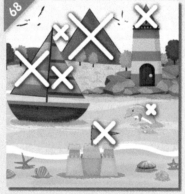

72

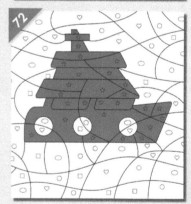

63

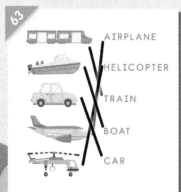

AIRPLANE
HELICOPTER
TRAIN
BOAT
CAR

69

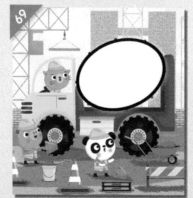

73

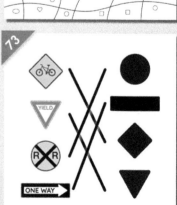

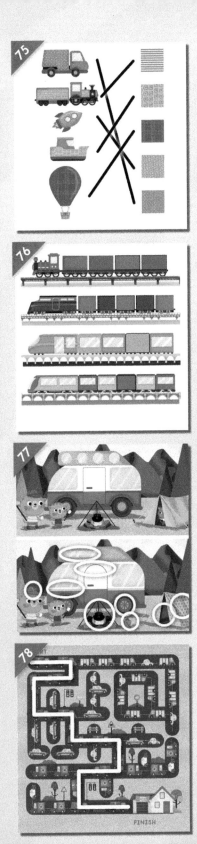

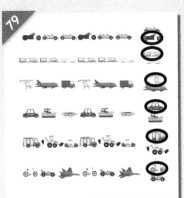

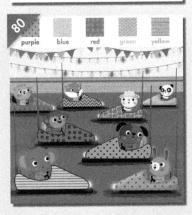

ABOUT THE AUTHOR

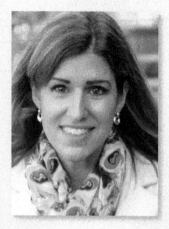

Valerie Deneen is the founder of InnerChildFun.com, where she writes about crafts, play ideas, and educational activities for kids of all ages. Valerie is a speaker, creative play advocate, brand ambassador, and active Rotarian. Her work has been featured in Highlights High Five, FamilyFun Magazine, PBS Parents, and various morning talk shows. For creative play ideas sent directly to your inbox, visit Valerie's blog at InnerChildFun.com and subscribe to the weekly newsletter.

ABOUT THE ILLUSTRATOR

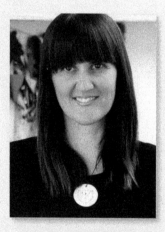

Rachael McLean is a children's book illustrator living in a lovely coastal town in Australia. Growing up by the sea, her days were filled with bright blue skies and hours whiled away drawing all kinds of cute characters in her sketchbook. These days her drawings spring to life from her trusty Wacom tablet, using a combination of Illustrator and Photoshop. Inspired by bright colors and all things whimsical, Rachael loves storytelling through her drawings and making people smile. Most days you'll find her with her rescue pups by her side and a nice cup of tea, making art and enjoying the best job in the world.